Contents

Acknowledgements

It has been a pleasure and a privilege to have worked on this project and through doing so to have had the opportunity to meet with a large number of people who have contributed in an equally large variety of ways.

The most important acknowledgements go to the young disabled people who have so generously and willingly participated in this project. Their contribution goes beyond the visible in that they have provided the underlying motivation and inspiration for the project (not to mention the fun along the way). I do not name these young people as some wish to remain anonymous. This work belongs to all of you.

I am grateful to the families, and friends of families, who have welcomed me into their homes and shared their lives so openly with me. It has been a delight to have had the opportunity to meet and work with you in this way.

Thanks also go to the different organisations that have made me so welcome and given of their time and resources. Whilst it is not possible to name the many individuals taking part, two organisations have made a large contribution to the project – many thanks, then, to 'Interplay' in Swansea and 'Out and About' in Ipswich. Not only did these organisations introduce me to groups of young disabled people, they also gave their ideas, their time and made me feel very much at home.

Thanks to the members of the loose-knit advisory group for their enthusiasm and positive criticisms of the project as it developed. A particular thank you goes to Linda Ward (who suggested I should do this work) and to Emma Stone from the Joseph Rowntree Foundation for 'being there' along the way.

A vote of thanks goes to my friend and colleague Claire Tregaskis who has acted as an advisory consultant to the project. Our many discussions about leisure have inevitably found their way into the 'flavour' of the report.

Thanks to Kyle Buxton for technical support and advice with the graphics and for creating the collages.

Finally, there is one person who although he died three years ago has nevertheless been very much a part of this project. Thanks, then, to my son Kim.

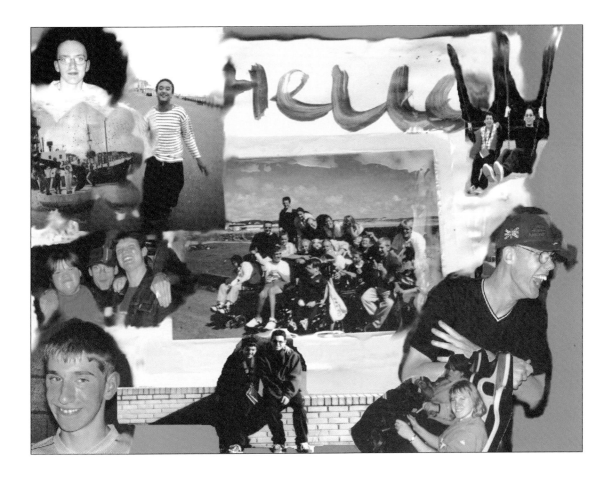

1 Introduction

Leisure is an important aspect of our lives allowing us to expand our horizons through the development of our interests, whilst at the same time giving us the opportunity to meet and interact with others holding similar interests. We are likely to make new friends through our leisure pursuits just as we are likely to spend our leisure time with established friends. In addition to giving us possibilities of developing relationships, leisure is recognised as giving us opportunities to follow our interests, to push ourselves to new physical, social and psychological limits. An important feature of our leisure time is that we have the opportunity to engage in activities that make us happy, so developing our self-esteem, confidence, emotional and psychological well-being.

Leisure takes on an additional significance for disabled people who generally do not experience an ease of access into mainstream education or work. Barriers to full and equal participation in these areas result in young disabled people both having more time for leisure pursuits whilst simultaneously experiencing greater difficulty in accessing leisure services, activities and pastimes (Aitchison, 2000; Petrie *et al.*, 2000). Leisure, therefore, is identified as a key area through which to build bridges towards the inclusion of young disabled people within the mainstream.

Definition of leisure

Throughout this project, leisure has been loosely defined as any chosen activity/pastime when not engaging with school, college, or paid employment. Thus, leisure time is viewed as: time spent at home when not doing schoolwork; watching television; reading; talking on the phone; using the computer; time spent at an after-school or holiday club; time spent in the gym; the cinema; the countryside; the nightclub; the coffee bar; on holiday; and, finally, time spent having a break from all activities – time spent doing nothing at all. Crucial to this definition is young disabled people being able to choose what they do, and when, where and with whom they do it. Such a wide definition allows leisure to be viewed as an integral part of the lives of young disabled people in contrast to being more narrowly defined as something provided in a particular venue. It has also allowed us to pose a question about 'missing' time – time when non-disabled young people are engaging in leisure pursuits of their choice and disabled young people are at home (usually without the company of friends) with their parents watching television or playing on the computer. Whilst such activities are common to all young people, many disabled young people appear to be spending a disproportionate amount of time engaging in such activities alone, at the same time as having fewer alternatives than non-disabled young people.

The context

This exploration of leisure, specifically 'access to inclusive leisure', is firmly placed within the context of recent legislation such as the Disability Discrimination Act, 1995; the Human Rights Act, 1998; and *Valuing People: A New Strategy for Learning Disability for the 21st Century* (HMSO, 2001). Policy initiatives such as the Quality Protects Programme (England), Children First (Wales) and the Framework for Social Justice (Scotland) all aim to bridge the gap between legislative aspirations and the daily experience of vulnerable young people. Such legislation and policy initiatives clearly state that disabled young people have the right to be included in the mainstream and that the move from provision that excludes to provision that includes is an essential aspect of a caring society:

> *People with learning disabilities often do not take part in ordinary leisure activities. Leisure is rarely built into individual or community care plans. It tends to be seen as an optional extra, generally coming well down the list of agencies'*

priorities when decisions are being made about resources. Enabling people to use a wider range of leisure opportunities can make a significant contribution to improving quality of life, can help to tackle social exclusion, and encourage healthy life styles.
(HMSO, 2001, para. 7.37, p. 80)

Many of the young disabled people taking part in this project had heard about the Disability Discrimination Act; few were familiar with Valuing People and the possibility of accessing Direct Payments; none were familiar with policy initiatives such as Quality Protects that seeks to bridge the gap between the legislative framework and the daily experience of disabled people. At the same time, many disabled young people were frustrated by the gap they perceived between the rhetoric of the legislation and their experience of exclusion. Not surprisingly, therefore, they were eager to be involved in a project that sought to make their experience visible. Within a short space of time, young disabled people identified the following areas as key to their inclusion in leisure pastimes, services and activities:

- friendships and relationships

- sharing of mutual experience

- information

- communication

- support

- redefinition of participation

- transport

- money.

3

The process

Whilst the project does not claim to be comprehensively inclusive, a serious attempt has been made to uncover the leisure experience of a wide variety of disabled young people, in as many different situations as possible. In keeping with an underlying philosophy of inclusion and empowerment, the project sought to offer an experience of being valued, respected, included and empowered to all young disabled people taking part. To this end, the project included young disabled people within their family setting as well as young disabled people within organisations. This allowed for the involvement of young disabled people presently excluded from both statutory and voluntary leisure services. In acknowledgement of the possible influence of age, geographic, ethnic and gender variables, participants include:

- the upper (16–19) and lower (12–15) ends of the age range

- young people from both urban and rural environments

- a diverse racial/ethnic mix

- males and females.

Finally, recognising the impact and effect that different impairments have on our experience, the project sought to include young people with as many different impairments as possible.

To this end, young people from four different projects (three in England and one in Wales) that provided a variety of leisure activities for disabled teenagers participated in the research. Three of the projects ran schemes for children and young people with specific impairments – one for young people with visual impairments and two for young people with learning difficulties – whilst the fourth project included young people with a wide variety of impairments. Young people from these projects chose their own level of involvement in the research – some choosing to give large amounts of time through a variety of means, others giving perhaps one interview or providing a photograph. In addition to the projects taking part, the research also involved five young people from within their family situation. Overall, approximately 100 young people (about an equal number of young men and young women) were directly involved. This sample included young people from minority ethnic backgrounds but did not include a group of young disabled people from a minority ethnic background. Professionals, ranging from project co-ordinators, development workers and support workers, also participated. In addition to those young people directly participating, the research also drew on the broad experience of six other projects – four in Scotland and two in England. Unfortunately, this project did not have the scope to follow through with an unsuccessful attempt to make links with young disabled people in Northern Ireland, although initial enquiries indicated additional barriers in accessing mainstream leisure services because of the long-standing political situation.

Being guided by young disabled people

In keeping with present recommendations that services are shaped by those people using them, the project was guided by the young people's experience, interest and their view of priorities. Viewing leisure in the context of the educational experience is one example of this. Prior to comments from young disabled people as to the way in which their experience of education impacted upon their experience of leisure, it had not been anticipated that the project would touch upon the world of education. One group of participants particularly keen to emphasise this connection has plans to present the findings of the final report to an invited local audience comprising educational professionals and leisure service providers.

Engaging with young disabled people, having fun ...

In whatever manner individuals or groups of young people participated in the project, an important prerequisite was that involvement in the project offered the opportunity of an enjoyable, positive and empowering experience. One example of the way this was achieved lies within an interview that took place between two young disabled men, both using facilitated communication. The (very ordinary) questions they chose to ask each other provided the starting point for an invaluable conversation giving insight into their particular experience. For the young men involved, the meeting provided the rare opportunity of spending time in a positive environment with someone else with a similar impairment. Reflecting upon the meeting, one of the young men stated:

> *I am very glad that I have been able to express myself in the way that I have, and feel that my consciousness has been raised by the experience.*

The meeting that took place was completely ordinary – what was extraordinary was the fact that neither of the young men had previously had such an opportunity. The occasion rendered undeniably visible the fact that the preoccupations of these two young men were similar to those of the majority of young people – friendships, music, education, exams, future prospects – in spite of their particular experience of exclusion. In many ways, their method of communication added to the depth of the dialogue as each word spelled out took great effort and was therefore carefully considered.

Flexibility of methods

In keeping with the aim that the project be as inclusive as possible, flexibility of approach was an important dynamic throughout. To this end, many different methods were used: semi-structured interviews, group discussions, peer interviews, observation, spending time with, attending 'Circle of support' meetings, chatting, engaging in leisure pursuits with, 'hanging out' with, telephone interviews, leisure diaries, drawings, photographs, art work with photographs, video recording, taped pieces *Big Brother* style (i.e. individuals talking directly into a tape on their own), poetry, writing and networking.

Photography and artwork

Some disabled young people perceived as having learning difficulties were not able to engage in conversations about their leisure experience. After several attempts to find meaningful ways to fully involve young people perceived as having learning difficulties in the project on their own terms (spending time with, engaging with other people known to them, observation), it was through work with photographs that some success was achieved. Photography and artwork provided a medium through which:

- the experience of people unable to articulate with language in any of its many shapes and forms could be directly conveyed to the reader

- the views of a group of disabled young people perceived as having learning difficulties could be fully included as an integral part of the project.

This particular area of the project raises more questions than it claims to answer – questions of an ethical nature (whilst names can be changed to protect confidentiality when using language, how can that same confidentiality be given when using photographs?; how do we highlight issues whilst protecting people's vulnerabilities?; when it is unclear as to whether the young people understand the nature of the research process, is it fair to gauge their consent through the fact that they are having a good time whilst producing the images?) in addition to questions arising in the analysis of such material. For the purposes of this report, two very simple rules of thumb were used when deciding on the use of images for publication:

1   All images show individuals and groups in a positive light.

2   Analysis is kept to a simple, straightforward level as, for example, in the image of the young girl singing, enclosed by a heart, flagged by the words, 'I love you. Steps'.

Bearing in mind such notes of caution around the use of photographs, however, the process provides evidence that the interests of young disabled people perceived as having learning difficulties are no different from those of other young people. In addition to this, it allowed some young people perceived as having learning difficulties to be meaningful participants in the project. It is hoped that future work will further explore the possibilities of working with images as a means of including young people on their own terms and of giving value to a medium through which young disabled people perceived as having learning difficulties might have the confidence to express themselves.

Consent

The issue of gaining the consent of young people was dealt with in several different ways:

•   Obtaining consent from parents of young people under the age of 16 and for all young people with learning difficulties.

•   Responding to the wishes of young people as they participated. For example, if someone showed they were not interested in engaging with an activity, their disinterest was taken as an indication that they did not want to participate at that particular point in time.

- Participants had the opportunity to see their contribution in the report format, before it reached the publication stage. Contributions were adjusted or withdrawn at this stage according to the wishes of participants.

Evolving practice

This project, spanning a period of nine months, was roughly divided into three stages:

1 an initial exploratory phase used to find out what was happening in different parts of the country

2 a concentrated phase of working with young disabled people individually, in groups, with organisations and/or families

3 producing the report alongside some of the young people involved in stage two.

There was a great enthusiasm from all to fully participate in and contribute towards the project. The isolation and disempowerment of young disabled people was mirrored by the isolation and a perceived lack of power from families, support workers, project workers and, on occasion, the projects themselves. It was therefore seen as important that involvement in the project was an enjoyable experience for individuals or groups in whatever role they happened to be playing in the lives of young disabled people.

Some of the young people taking part have chosen to protect their identity by remaining anonymous whilst others have chosen to use their own names. The report reflects these different choices.

At the beginning of the project, it was envisaged that the research might include an exploration of facilities (such as leisure centres); sporting activities; arts and cultural activities. Such explorations were, however, placed on a back burner as the young people unanimously told of their experiences from a slightly different perspective. In order to acknowledge developments in these areas, a 'resource list' has been included at the end of the report. This list gives contact details of organisations seeking to give young disabled people opportunities to participate in mainstream sporting, artistic and cultural activities. These organisations work in very different ways – some providing workshops to projects working in the wider area of leisure provision. It is hoped that this list will be used by voluntary and statutory organisations keen to give young disabled people new leisure experiences.

2 Talking about leisure led to talks about everything else

Talking with young people about what they liked to do in their time out of school/college quickly led to conversations about all sorts of things. At an early stage in the research, it became obvious that young people were making links between different parts of their lives that traditional (adult-led) research does not allow for. Leisure was not seen in isolation from other aspects of their lives, forming as it did an integral part of their daily experience. The young people involved in this project overwhelmingly saw leisure as either 'hanging out' with other people or 'doing things' with people they enjoyed to be with. Leisure, therefore, was primarily defined as being about mutually enjoyable relationships.

Whether the conversation was through language, photographs, drawing, or 'spending time with', the constant themes were those of friendships and communication; having fun with other people; making choices and being present. There was, as there is for all teenagers, a tension between dependence and independence; becoming an adult and remaining a child; having adventures out of the reach of responsible adults and returning to the safe familiarity of home. In short, conversations with young disabled people about leisure led to conversations about growing up, leaving home, sitting exams, reflecting upon childhood, family, friends, sexual relationships, school, work, college, holidays, money and future aspirations. The stories being told were the preoccupations of the majority of teenagers in the UK in 2001.

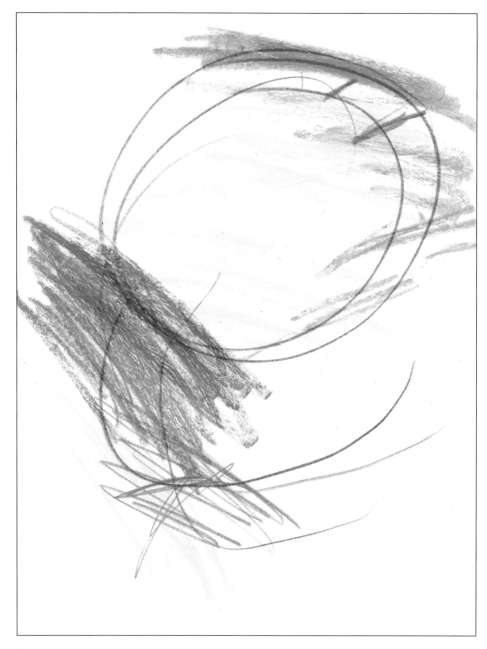

Leisure, therefore, was primarily defined as being about mutually enjoyable relationships.

Whilst impairment makes little difference to teenage concerns, it does make a difference to their experiences and the way in which others treat them. The majority of teenagers involved in this project live with impairments of one sort or another and as a result have in common the experience of their lives being marked by an assumption that there is 'something wrong' with them. Consequently, young disabled people describe their lives as being tainted by the experience of exclusion. All the young people able to articulate through language chose to tell of their painful experiences of exclusion – exclusion from schools, examination systems, communities, everyday activities, friendships and ordinary relationships. Listening to others talk about the lives of those young people unable to express themselves through language, spending time with such young people told that same story of exclusion and isolation. A clear message emerging from the telling of these stories is that, as adults, predominantly non-disabled adults, we are not used to listening to the voices of young disabled people. On several occasions during the project, while groups of disabled young people sat and talked about their lives, professionals known to them came close and listened, fascinated by the way in which they were expressing themselves. Afterwards, they told how they had never heard such detail about the lives of the young people before, even those they considered to know well. They confessed they had no idea of the painful nature of the experiences of exclusion and had never before heard the articulate passion with which the young people told their stories.

The young people involved in this project want their stories to be told; it is their hope that in doing this they will help other younger disabled teenagers and children to have a better experience and that their own experience of exclusion will change.

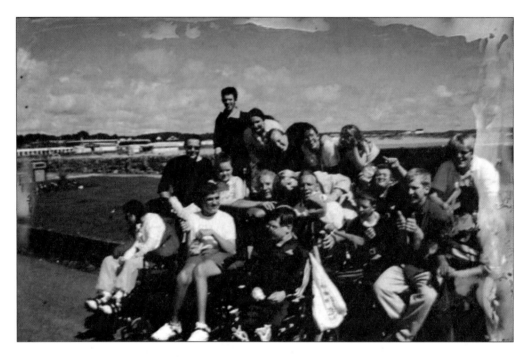

The young people involved in this project want their stories to be told.

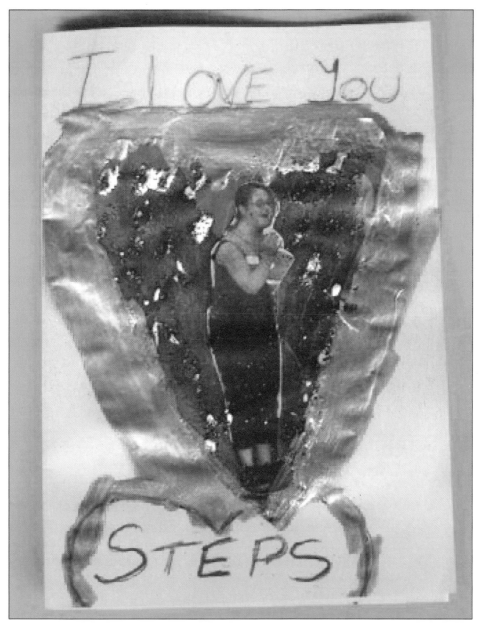

The stories being told were the preoccupations of the majority of teenagers in the UK in 2001.

3 Definitions

What do we mean by 'inclusion'?

The response of the majority of young disabled people to the questions on the subject of 'inclusive leisure' was to talk about relationships. However, the same subject put to non-disabled young people evoked a variety of responses. The response of one non-disabled teenager sums up the way many understand the term:

> *I'm not the best person to ask about this. It doesn't have anything to do with me. That's for disabled people isn't it?*

Conversations with service providers, project leaders and support staff showed a similar understanding: 'inclusive' leisure is widely understood to be something that is done to and for disabled people. There was little evidence to show that 'inclusive' leisure is understood as something that affects all of us. Consequently, there does not appear to be a wide understanding that the inclusion of young disabled people into the mainstream would be of benefit to everyone. There was further confusion from projects providing leisure activities for disabled young people. ' Inclusive leisure' variously meant:

- giving young disabled people a choice

- disabled young people participating, as a group or individually, in mainstream leisure activities and facilities

- including non-disabled brothers and sisters in segregated play-schemes

- providing opportunities to meet new challenges in a 'safe' (segregated) setting in order to enable young disabled people to try these out in their local, mainstream settings

- providing one-to-one support for young disabled people to take part in activities of their choice in their community.

What do we mean by 'leisure'?

Whereas for young disabled people leisure is about having a good time, being with people they want to be with, there appears to be a different agenda for service providers who view leisure opportunities, particularly those aimed at young people with learning difficulties, as an opportunity to 'learn' and 'develop skills'. For example, one youth project is designed to provide not only choice in leisure activities for disabled teenagers but also an emphasis on 'developing life skills'. Similarly, a personal assistant project, concerned about the lack of access to mainstream leisure for young people attending a special school, describes its aims as follows:

- to create a safe learning environment

- to establish what real and informed choices are

- to develop group work skills

- to develop social skills relevant to mainstream opportunities

- to develop the self-esteem and confidence of the group

- to equip the young people with the necessary skills to recruit and use personal assistants

- to recruit some peer educators from the group.

Another vacation scheme offering adventure holidays to groups of young people with a visual impairment sought to:

- increase personal independence

- improve social skills

- meet new challenges in a safe supportive environment

- gain confidence in a range of leisure activities to enable them to access mainstream leisure services at home.

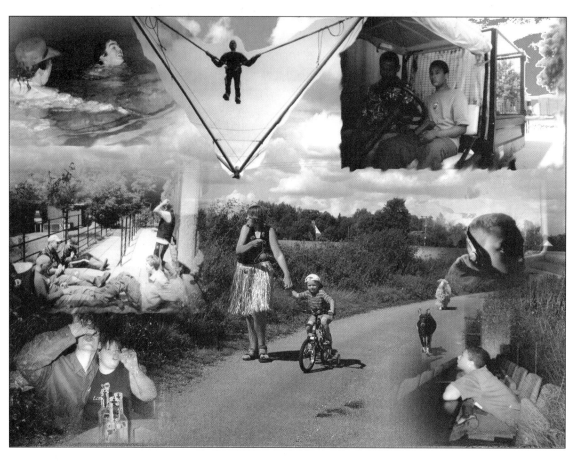

… for young disabled people leisure is about having a good time, being with the people they want to be with.

What do young disabled people think?

The young people taking part in this project want to be able to access the same opportunities as all young people. They are less interested in defining terms than in 'getting things right'. In this sense, inclusive leisure is not something that takes place in a particular building, at a particular time, with particular people. Inclusive leisure is viewed as a process through which we all belong in whatever setting we happen to be in. Therefore, inclusive leisure is viewed as something that happens in the swimming pool, the nightclub, shopping centres, at home, in the park, in the playground, the pub, the beach, the art gallery, etc. Young people overwhelmingly see leisure as either 'hanging out' with other people or 'doing things' with people they enjoy being with. Leisure, therefore, is primarily defined as being about mutually enjoyable relationships. In this definition, inclusive leisure is not confined to one particular place; rather, it is seen as a natural process through which all of us can go to the places we want to go to, with the people we want to be with. Such a definition carries within it the potential for the breakdown of all exclusive barriers – impairment, age, gender, race, ethnicity, class and religion.

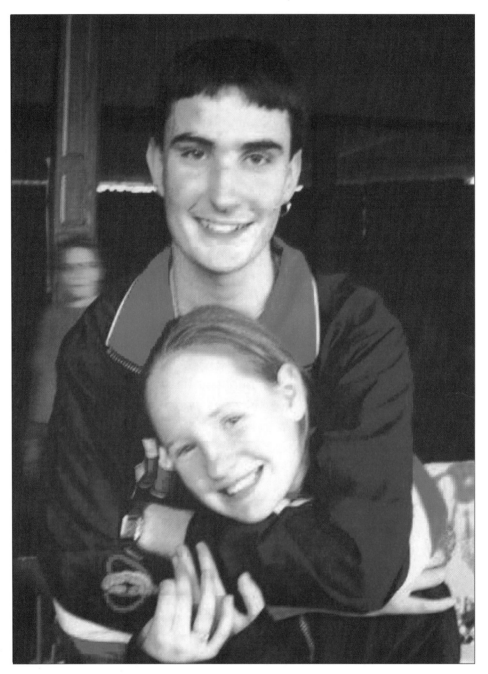

... inclusive leisure is seen as a natural process through which all of us can go to the places we want to go to, with the people we want to be with.

4 Redefining terms

Independence

In order to engage with inclusive leisure as defined by young disabled people, it is necessary to think about key concepts such as independence and participation. Traditionally, independence is seen as 'doing something on one's own'. Such a definition excludes many and falsely implies that we operate in isolation from one another. What the young disabled people involved in this project wanted was the opportunity to stretch themselves to their limits – whatever those limits happen to be. Whenever appropriate support was used to support this goal, the young people showed no indication that requiring support was a negative thing. On the contrary, the presence of appropriate support allowed for new adventures to take place.

There were several examples of schemes supporting young disabled people for a short amount of time in mainstream leisure activities of their choosing. At the end of the specified time, it was expected that the young person would not require support to participate in the sessions. Young disabled people who, because of their impairment, were not able to achieve such independence were either denied the opportunity to participate in such schemes or seen to fail if they did not achieve independence. In order for these young people to be fully included, to have their presence valued, the concept of 'interdependence' needs to be recognised, valued and allowed to replace the present concept of 'independence'.

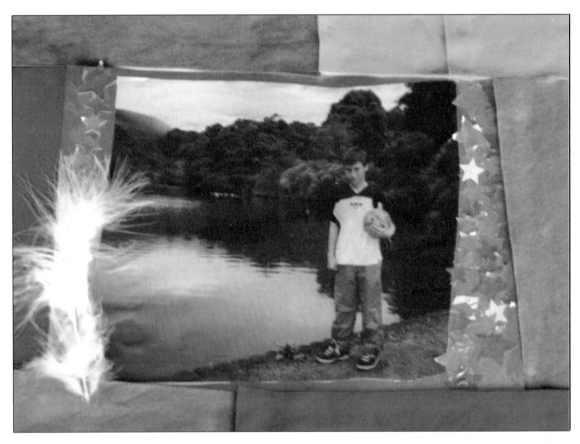

What the young disabled people involved in this project wanted was the opportunity to stretch themselves to their limits ...

Participation

Similarly, it is necessary to examine our ideas about 'participation'. Some of the young people taking part in this project were unable to participate in activities and yet showed that they were clearly pleased to be present. Young disabled people and their parents told of their experiences of going to organisations such as Guides, Scouts and Woodcraft Folk. Often, if an individual did not 'join in', their presence would be questioned. In such cases, participation is seen as 'doing something' rather than 'being somewhere'. Young disabled people, however, appeared to see things slightly differently. Some of them showed (perhaps through their body language or their behaviour) that they were pleased to be in places, even if they could not actively take part in what was going on. If such pleasure to be present was accompanied by other people positively welcoming their presence, it appeared that participation was in place. In this way, then, participation was defined as an individual enjoying being present at the same time as others welcoming their presence. Participation was therefore placed within the realms of relationship. Such a definition – participation as positive interaction between people – opens the door to a very different experience for young disabled people presently perceived as being 'unable to participate'. It also allows for increasing the possibilities of the building of relationships between disabled and non-disabled young people. Just as disabled young people need the opportunity to be present, so, too, do non-disabled young people require their presence if they are to learn that impairment is an ordinary part of human life.

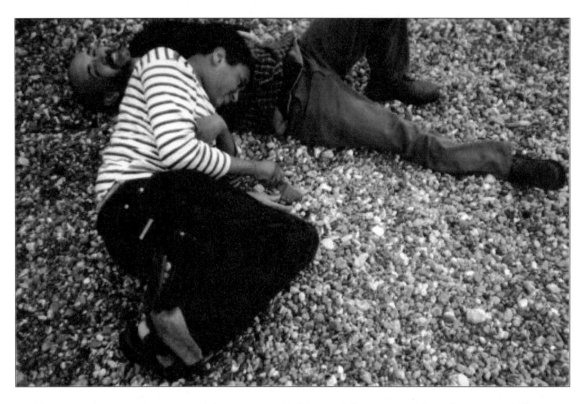

... the presence of appropriate support allowed for new adventures to take place.

5 Relationship

Although there was great enthusiasm for trying out new leisure activities, it appeared that, generally, activities were seen as secondary to the possibility of either making new friends or spending time with established friends. Throughout the project, talks about leisure with young disabled people rapidly led to talks about their educational experience – school being the place where most young people make friends.

Making a link between education and leisure

The experience of social exclusion and the accompanying social isolation was familiar to all the young disabled people taking part in this project. Many described this isolation as stemming from their educational experiences – whether they attended a mainstream or a segregated school. As school is the main opportunity for children and young people to make friends and learn about relationships, it is perhaps not surprising that a strong link was being made between leisure opportunities and educational experience. Young people who had experienced both segregated and mainstream schools explained how both types of schools set them apart and in doing so created barriers to the building of friendships. As one young man who has attended both segregated and mainstream schools said, 'Mainstream schools treat you differently to the other students', whilst at the same time, 'It's a bit harder being out in the real world after special school'.

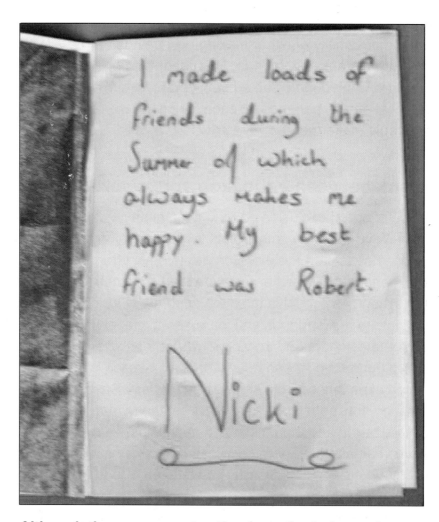

I made loads of friends during the Summer of which always makes me happy. My best friend was Robert.

Nicki

Although there was great enthusiasm for trying out new leisure activities, it appeared that, generally, activities were seen as secondary to the possibility of either making new friends or spending time with established friends.

Those young disabled people who attended segregated schools generally went to school outside of their neighbourhood and consequently often lived some distance from their school friends. The only times young people in this situation were likely to see each other were in segregated settings, at after-school clubs, in holiday schemes or specialist youth clubs. The isolation of only children attending segregated schools was particularly pronounced.

The majority of young people perceived as having learning difficulties (generally, this group appeared more likely than disabled young people with other impairments to attend segregated schools) spoke about their family as being their best friends, the people they most liked to do things with. This stands in sharp contrast to other young people taking part in the research who said, as the majority of teenagers do, that they were 'fed up with family' and wanted to be with groups of young people, doing the things that young people traditionally do. An important part of the teenage experience is 'trying things out'. Not only are disabled young people socially isolated, they are also being denied ordinary teenage opportunities to learn about the world.

Attendance at a mainstream school, whilst seen by the majority of disabled young people to be preferable, did not necessarily make things any easier in that it produced a different experience of isolation. Many of the disabled young people attending local mainstream schools found that they were constantly being 'left out', made to feel different, socially isolated and sometimes physically bullied. This experience in school had a great influence on time spent out of school, as some young people quite simply did not have any friends. Both Lizzie and Ben spoke about their experience of the few non-disabled friends they did have, suffering abuse from the larger group. Lizzie said that she knew 'she had a real friend' when that person stood up for her against the majority group. Ben talked about his younger sister being bullied simply because she was his sister. Being without friends means that there is no one apart from family with whom to go to the swimming pool, go into town, sit in cafes or hang out in parks with. Hence, some young people felt strongly that the quality of time spent out of school depended on relationships with other young people in school.

For some young people taking part, the time spent in school was the only time they spent with other people their own age apart from their brothers or sisters.

Whilst some young people had relationships with their peers in school, often they were unable to spend time with these friends out of school. This was something reported by those young people attending a 'resourced unit' within a mainstream school. Just as those young people attending segregated school had to travel out of their community to get to school, so, too, did the young people attending resourced units. Any friends made at school usually live some distance away. Because of this, this group of young disabled people are unlikely to spend time with their school friends when they are out of school.

A further barrier to developing friendships was described by young people requiring 'one-to-one' support. The presence of a support worker not only inhibited friendships but also on occasions caused resentment, as other young people wanted time without adults who they saw to be in a supervisory role.

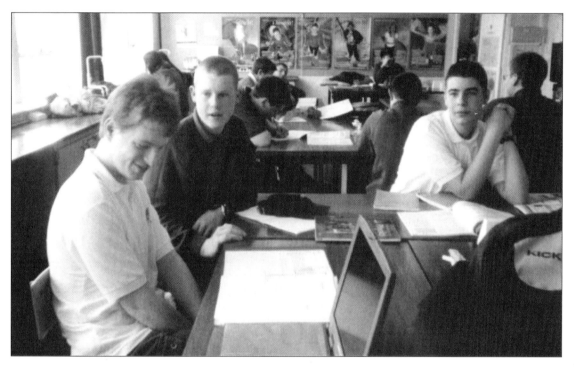

... some young people felt strongly that the quality of time spent out of school depended on relationships with other young people in school.

6 Are the barriers always the same, no matter what the impairment?

Although all the young people involved in this project told of their experience of being excluded from mainstream leisure activities, as the project developed, it emerged that the barriers to living ordinary lives facing young people with impairments varied slightly depending on the nature of the impairment. Such differences need to be acknowledged if services are to provide good quality, appropriate support to young disabled people. A lack of making distinctions in this way leads to certain barriers to participation being rendered invisible. When barriers are made invisible, the onus is put back on the problem lying with the individual with impairment. An example of this was a young man with a visual impairment and learning difficulties on a holiday scheme for young people with visual impairments. This young man was set apart from the others on the scheme 'because of his learning difficulties'. Because his individual support needs had not been taken into account, both he and the other young people were learning the lesson that 'he did not fit in', 'was not one of them', because of his impairment. Had appropriate support been in place, all the young people would have had the opportunity to experience an environment in which impairment was not a reason for exclusion. In contrast to this, on another occasion, a young man with a hearing impairment who used a range of communication strategies including British Sign Language (BSL) had the support of a communication worker fluent in BSL during his time out with a group of young people with a mix of different impairments. Such support enabled him to be part of the group.

In looking at this issue, it is important to note that any difference in treatment has more to do with the perceptions others have of particular impairments than with the impairment itself. Although the following section by no means covers the experience of all barriers affecting all types of impairment (notably absent are the experiences of young people with hearing impairments), some of the barriers arising for those young disabled people taking part in this project are explored.

Barriers facing young people with learning difficulties

Disabled young people perceived as having learning difficulties were much less likely to have non-disabled friends than young people with physical or sensory impairments. This meant that their opportunities for going out with friends to take part in mainstream leisure activities, activities so easily taken for granted by non-disabled young people, were markedly more limited. In addition to this, it also appeared to be more difficult for young disabled people perceived as having learning difficulties to have relationships with each other independently from adults. This was owing partly to the fact that the support levels for young disabled people perceived as having learning difficulties are likely to be higher, partly perhaps owing to the effects of impairment and partly also to a particular element of the relationship between non-disabled adults and young people with learning difficulties. There was a marked tendency for adults to be very protective towards young disabled people perceived as having learning difficulties and an associated lack of confidence from the young people to 'have a go'. This resulted in the majority of disabled young people perceived as having learning difficulties looking to support workers for friendship rather than engaging directly with other young people – disabled or non-disabled, whether or not they were perceived as having learning difficulties. This was particularly noticeable for both young women and for young people from minority ethnic backgrounds perceived as having learning difficulties. This means that young women from minority ethnic backgrounds are likely to be particularly isolated because of the interplay of discriminatory factors affecting ethnicity, gender and impairment.

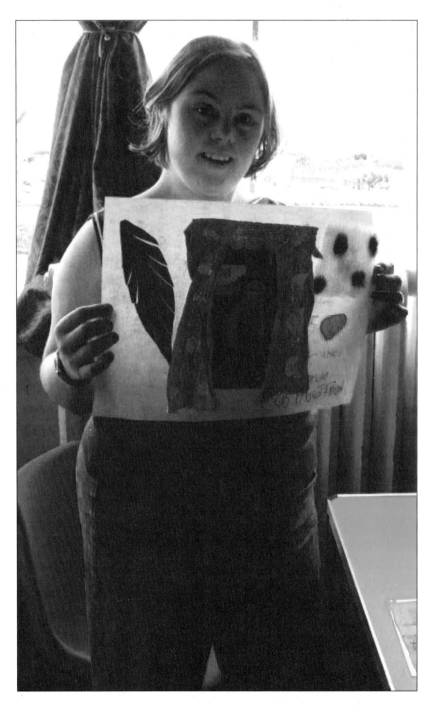

Just as young people perceived as having learning difficulties are not used to expressing themselves freely, nor are we used to taking their views, hence their lives, seriously.

The socially conditioned lack of confidence on the part of young disabled people perceived as having learning difficulties means that there are barriers for them to overcome in finding whether or not they have preferences, what their opinion is or in being able to say what they want. Just as young people perceived as having learning difficulties are not used to expressing themselves freely, nor are we used to taking their views, hence their lives, seriously.

Barriers facing young people with visual impairments

In the same way that the barriers to full participation for young people perceived as having learning difficulties were unique to them because of the way in which their impairment was viewed, so, too, did young people with visual impairments tell of particular barriers they commonly faced. This group of young people told of major difficulties in going out independently.

> *Other people are making life harder for me like when I go shopping people do not look where they are going so they bump into me.*

Mita's experience was reflected by other young people with a visual impairment who reported difficulty in finding their way about town because of the fact that shops were constantly changing the layout of their displays, few escalators or stairs had their edges marked out, and print on signs and labels was almost always too small to read. Asking for help in situations sometimes led to the building of relationships but at other times meant being treated with extreme rudeness and disrespect. Sally told how she regularly had problems with taxi drivers who dropped her off at the wrong place and drove off leaving her stranded. Matthew told how his experience of going out on his own depended on who he happened to meet and the way in which they responded to him. He reported on some occasions being treated with great kindness, whilst on others he felt people were offended by his presence. It is a sad reflection on our deeply segregated society that he was recently asked by a young child sitting near to him on the bus, 'Do you eat?'

As with the majority of young disabled people taking part in this project, young people with visual impairments were able to identify areas of difficulty in their lives, discriminating between the effects of impairment and unnecessary disabling barriers:

In my free time I like to play the computer, watch TV, read books, play cards and go shopping with someone. Most of the time I like doing these things with a friend. I find going shopping the hardest because of a number of reasons which are listed below:

1 *I have major problems seeing some of the steps because most of them are not marked in a different colour so I am sometimes afraid to go down them.*

2 *Some shopping centres do not have stairs or lifts so I find it very difficult to go up escalators because I cannot see when to get off and on them and if someone else tells me they do not tell me quick enough.*

3 *Some people do not look where they are going so they bump into me and I can easily fall over so I always have to be with someone when I go out.*

I do not play the computer very often because I have real problems seeing the arrow and sometimes the print on the internet is too small for me to read.

I have the same problems reading books because most of the books I want to read have very small print so I don't really enjoy reading very many books but I do not have any difficulties watching TV or playing cards.

After I lost my eyesight I have always wished to do lots of things that I cannot do and every time I look at a person that has got their eyesight and is doing things that they want to do so I wish I was like them.

Here are a list of things I want to do but I cannot do:

1 Go outside and play games with my friends without help.

2 Going shopping on my own and buying what I want and being able to see how much they cost by myself without anyone having to tell me.

3 Make my own breakfast, lunch and dinner without help from other people.

Several young disabled people with visual impairments spoke of the social exclusion they experienced as the result of being unable to read new and popular books – Harry Potter was the example given – at the same time as everyone else. As they had to wait until the book was produced in large print, by which time everyone else had stopped talking about it, they had been unable to participate in discussions at the time when the majority of their friends had been reading it. There were some books that they were never able to read, as they are not produced in large print, Braille or on tape. Mita also brought up the point that, because she was not able to access large-print school texts, she was unable to keep up with her peers in class. Such exclusion was felt keenly by the young people and had an adverse effect on their relationships with non-disabled teenagers.

Barriers facing young people with communication impairments

The dominance of speech and language as the principal form of communication means that young people who cannot easily access speech and/or language are greatly disadvantaged in their opportunities for building relationships. Generally, these barriers arise as the result of the speed with which most of us communicate through language; a lack of awareness and sensitivity to different methods of communication; and the lack of recognition of communication support as a priority support need. Even within the educational setting, where communication support is most likely to be provided, young people told of major barriers they experienced in having their communication recognised and therefore their support needs met:

Osian: *I was taught at school by my speech therapist to do facilitated communication at school and I did it with everyone and then I went into the leavers' class and they didn't want to do it with me but they said that I wouldn't co-operate and I was so angry that I refused to communicate with anyone including the speech therapist because she backed up the staff.*

Mother: *Shall I add something?*

Osian: *Yes.*

Mother: *School had been taught how to do facilitated communication. School learnt. Then Osian went into the leavers' class and it's clear that they do not want to do it and when I go into school they discourage me from doing it. School says that head of class was untrained. Osian wrote a letter to school saying how unhappy he is about it. School said that the standard of the letter was much higher than communication produced at school. We showed them a video we have of Osian communicating at home, but it didn't make any difference. They did not believe that Osian could communicate.*

For young people whose first language was not English, the barriers were even greater. This arose as an issue for some Welsh-speaking young disabled people, as well as for young disabled people from minority ethnic backgrounds throughout the UK.

Young disabled people who do not use language to communicate were further disadvantaged, as their 'unconventional' methods of communication are even less likely to be recognised – for example, young disabled people dependent on others to 'read' their behaviour, body language, facial expression, sounds, their own signing system, finger spelling, touch, etc. It is fascinating to note the many different, endlessly creative ways young disabled people with communication impairments are finding to convey their preferences. For these young people, the lack of value placed on their expressive communication and the consequent lack of acknowledgement of that communication provides an insurmountable barrier to the building of relationships. For some young people taking part, the only place their communication was reliably and consistently acknowledged, understood and responded to was in their home.

Barriers facing young people with physical impairments

Young people with physical impairments told of their experience of the barriers to building relationships and their reduced possibilities of inclusion within the mainstream as the result of both ignorant and/or hostile attitudes and a lack of physical access. In this way, gaining access to public transport was a major frustration, as was their experience of being teased and bullied. Whilst the experience of not being able to physically access buildings was problematic, more hurtful was the general perception that they were different from others and consequently excluded from situations and relationships non-disabled young people take for granted. Young people with physical impairments were painfully aware of the ways in which their lives differed from their non-disabled peers – their additional difficulties in making friends; accessing transport; finding employment; going out; exploring their sexuality; moving primary relationships from family to friends; leaving home; going to all the places their non-disabled friends could take for granted; sitting exams; and 'being a teenager'. Perhaps because some of these young people had some access to relationships within the mainstream, they were aware of the subtleties of exclusion – the ways in which they would be picked last in PE at school; the ways they were often at the receiving end of tasteless jokes; the ways in which their family and friends would be picked upon because of their close relationships; and the ways in which, although they might have easier access to the mainstream than other young disabled people, they could never take such access for granted. In this sense, it becomes very difficult for young people with physical impairments to fully relax when they are out – although they often have pleasant and uneventful times, there is always the potential of hostile attitudes towards impairment coming their way or insurmountable physical barriers prohibiting access.

Barriers facing young disabled people perceived as having complex impairments and high support needs

For young people with complex impairments and high support needs, the issues are not so much about the details of what happens to them in the 'outside world' but rather about their right to be present in that world. Because of their extreme exclusion, young people perceived in this way can teach us much, not just about their own lives, but also about the process of inclusion. One young man perceived as having complex impairments and high support needs puts his constant rejection by the majority down to a widespread fear and dread of impairment:

> *Impairment is an ordinary part of human life but it is feared by so many, and I remind people of their fear.*

Are the barriers always the same, no matter what the impairment?

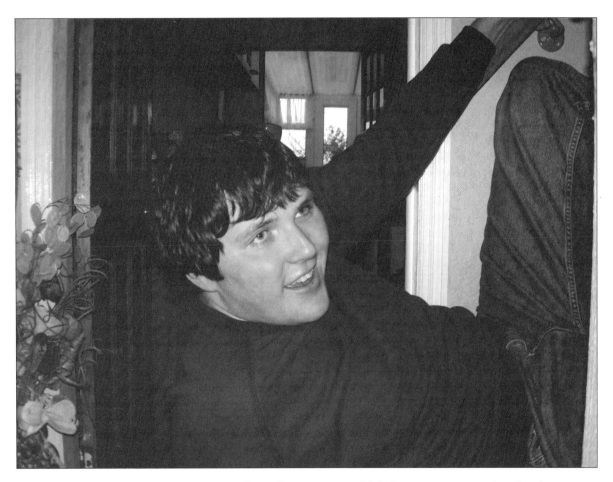

For young people with complex impairments and high support needs, the issues are not so much about the details of what happens to them in the 'outside world' but rather about their right to be present in that world.

From such a perspective, the biggest barrier facing the inclusion of such young people lies in the fact that we have not yet learned how to listen to them and to act on what we learn because we are not willing to face up to our own vulnerabilities.

Osian has been isolated all his life. Having attended a segregated school, and now attending a specialist day centre for people perceived to be autistic, he has no friends of his own age outside this setting. Osian's housing situation further exacerbates his exclusion – he lives in a small London flat where there is not enough room for him to see people separately from the rest of his family. Osian communicates beautifully and articulately through 'facilitated communication' – pointing out letters on a letter board. He knows exactly what he wants to do and where he wants to go. This communication was ignored by the social workers planning his future at the time of transition from children to adult services. Workers at the day centre are learning to facilitate Osian. Outside of the day centre, the only person able to facilitate Osian's communication is his mother. Osian has much to say on the subject of leisure, naturally placing it in the context of human rights:

> *I want to write about my leisure time and about my opportunities for enjoyment with other young people of my age. I am severely autistic and so need my mother with me at all times. I want this to change and I am sure that someone else would be able to take me to the places I frequent at the moment. I am worried that it is exhausting for her as she is getting older and I am very energetic.*

> *I want to find people who will take me ice skating, climbing and trampolining. I need people who will learn my method of communication which is facilitated communication, and I sadly feel that I am too isolated at present. I am at a wonderful day centre but after I come home I am alone with my parents.*

I am awfully in need of alternative sources of support. I am also pleased to say that I can type alone now but need more facilitators for validation purposes. I think that people are doubtful of my abilities because I am autistic but I am as articulate as the next man. However, I need the reassurance of a trained facilitator who can rescue me if my motor problems overwhelm me, which happens if I am tired or unwell.

I am awfully dependent in my impaired state, but it is made worse by a culture which has little value for a person who cannot stand up on his own two feet. I can stand in the literal sense but I need help with my communication, and I am appalled that my dependent state is seen as a reason for my being killed as a foetus if the defect had been known before I was born.

I think that I have something to offer other people, in that I am lacking some of their cynicism and sophisticated attitudes, which often mask an ignorance of the essential aspirations that should be the first preoccupations of all people.

People have forgotten the importance of simple qualities such as kindness and self-sacrifice for those weaker than themselves, and that there is a moral superiority in a person who perceives such needs, and is prepared to put themselves out to help an impaired fellow member of the human race. I am waiting to find such people and then I will take off and soar like a bird.

Barriers facing young disabled people requiring medical support

Generally speaking, there was little evidence of young disabled people requiring the availability of medical support being present in any of the leisure projects participating in the research. Whilst this was probably due to a variety of reasons, perhaps because of the nature of their medical condition – feeling unwell, being tired, etc.; or because individual support was relatively unusual; and/or due to a general reluctance to support young people with chronic medical conditions – their absence was conspicuous. The one exception to this was a young man attending a week-long activity scheme for disabled teenagers. Advertised as offering an experience of 'inclusive leisure', the scheme in fact was isolated and made up entirely of young disabled teenagers and support workers with little engagement with the wider community. The young man requiring medical support was further isolated as he could attend only when his support worker (arranged and paid for by his parents) was available. He therefore arrived later than the other young people and was positioned apart from them during the session.

There is little doubt that for all disabled teenagers, regardless of impairment, opportunities to 'try things out', to 'explore life', to have ordinary teenage adventures, to 'soar like a bird' are severely curtailed by the perceptions of non-disabled people in a disabling world.

7 What about the parents?

The teenage years are notorious for the difficulties they bring in negotiating new roles and identities within the family setting. Throughout the many conversations with young disabled people, I was struck by their mature attitude when they talked about their family relationships. Perhaps because of the frequency with which they had to negotiate their way through difficult issues within relationships, perhaps because of their enforced dependency on their parents, young disabled people appeared to be negotiating ordinary difficulties between young people and their parents with great skill. During the course of the project, it was common to hear professionals involved in providing leisure activities for disabled young people talk of the 'problem' of parents. What was generally meant by this was that parents are often perceived as being over-protective, unwilling to 'let go' of their teenage son or daughter. Disabled young people able to articulate on this subject, whilst agreeing that their parents sometimes worried about them too much, understood why this was the case. They thought it was reasonable for their parents to worry (all of them had had very unpleasant experiences), but were keen to work out ways of being able to go out, to stay out late, to take part in ordinary teenage experiences. Whilst such negotiations are all an ordinary part of growing up, the provision of good quality, appropriate, creative and flexible support would do much to facilitate the changing relationship between young disabled teenagers and their parents. Amidst the stories of 'over-protectiveness' were accounts from young disabled people – accounts illustrating the very ordinary nature of their relationship with their parents:

Even though we thought that we'd done a pretty thorough job on the cleaning, the parents still found time to follow round behind us and find fault upon their arrival for the return journey home. Oh well, what can you do?!

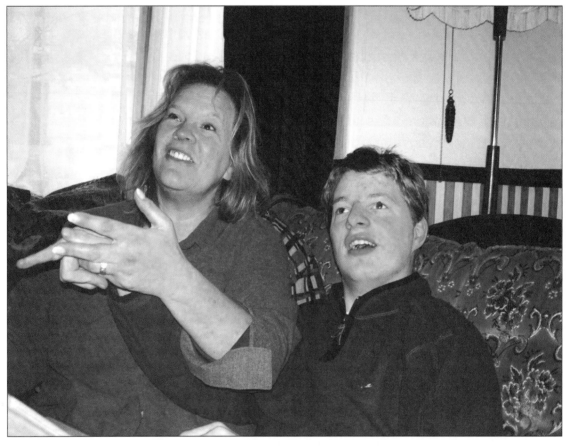

... the provision of good quality, appropriate, creative and flexible support would do much to facilitate the changing relationship between young disabled teenagers and their parents.

All too often, family relationships are considered outside the wider context of living with the complex issues of impairment and disablement. Positive, ordinary family relationships, with all the conflicting emotions they carry, can provide a springboard from which young disabled people are equipped to deal with the difficulties they inevitably face in a disabling world.

8 Young disabled people identify possible solutions – issues of support

Whilst young disabled people understood that barriers took many different forms – physical, attitudinal, economic, social, cultural and emotional – they were also clear that small things would make an enormous difference to their ability to keep abreast with mainstream culture and therefore enable them to be on an equal footing with their non-disabled peers. Along with many, Sally found her mobile phone invaluable as it enabled her to rearrange transport whilst out; keep in touch with her mother when she was running late; and make spontaneous arrangements with her friends. Matthew, too, is clear about the small things that make a difference to his experience of going out:

> *For the first time ever when I have travelled on my own I was asked, upon buying my ticket, whether I would like assistance when getting off the train at Peterborough. This was all arranged and as I am rather squeamish around train stations, I was also helped onto the train at Stevenage and placed near to a buffet car.*

The solutions offered up by young disabled people were, on the whole, modest, simple and relatively inexpensive. Access to appropriate support was seen by disabled young people as a major factor in enabling them, in some cases, to access mainstream activities, in others, to be present in their communities. Several themes on the issue of support emerged – transport, money, personal assistance, physical support, communication support, medical support and the support to facilitate friendships. The denial of any or all of these types of support forced young disabled people into an increasing, rather than a decreasing, dependency on their parents. At present, family members are most likely to be filling these support needs, as well as they can, within their own means and circumstances. As the teenage years are generally a time when young people become less, rather than more, dependent upon their parents, this gives disabled young people a different, more isolated, experience from that of the majority of teenagers.

Transport

I can't always do the things I like, because I always need someone with me and I don't have transport.

As is the case for teenagers generally, transport emerged as an issue affecting the lives of many disabled young people. This was particularly true for those young people living in rural areas. Because public transport is usually physically inaccessible, unwelcoming and does not take people from 'door to door', it can be very difficult for disabled young people to go out. For those disabled young people who are able to, learning to drive as early as possible is seen to be a very desirable option. Many disabled young people rely upon their families, usually their mother or their father, to take them to places.

In addition to the physical barriers of public transport, some young disabled people are made unwelcome by the way in which other people behave towards them. A support worker described her bus journey with one young man:

Paying to get on the bus, I felt the bus driver thought Kevin was a naughty, maybe even rude, boy that was out of my control and as a result of this the bus driver was rude to me when I asked the price of the journey. When it was time to get off the bus, Kevin wanted to talk to the driver who ignored him leaving me to explain the bus driver needed to concentrate on his driving and couldn't talk to him.

Later in the same day, Kevin and his support worker had the following experience:

Once again, when we got off the bus, Kevin wanted to talk to the bus driver. He also tried to touch the buttons. In an effort to stop Kevin touching the buttons, the bus driver grabbed his arm and pushed it away. In doing so Kevin's arm got bashed against the cash tin. The bus driver apologised to me, not Kevin, saying he had to do that as the buttons could not be touched by anyone but him. When we got off the bus, Kevin was looking at his arm and stroking it. I asked him if it hurt. He did not reply and started chatting about the cafe in the park so we went off to find it.

Older teenagers similarly face difficulties in organising their transport needs. Whilst on holiday together, a group of young disabled teenagers found a local taxi firm that supplied an accessible mini-bus that met their needs. Unfortunately, this service was not available after 4.00 p.m. Like most teenagers on holiday, this group generally started their day round about lunchtime; a taxi at 4.00 p.m. might get them out but would not get them back again. On one occasion, an easy journey back to the caravan turned into an 'event':

All was going well, that is until we tried to get back to the caravan park. We found that our minibus driver had gone home and after trying three other taxi companies in order to get a minibus (unfortunately being unsuccessful), we booked three taxis. The reason why we did this was because we worked under the assumption that a single taxi could only hold one wheelchair. So the first two taxis arrived and everyone other than Philip got back to the caravan park. After talking with one of the taxi drivers, I had discovered that he had cancelled the third taxi off his own back without our warning and this left Philip stranded. Although the fact remains that we got Philip back eventually, I did not like being taken for a fool just because I didn't know that a car could hold up to two folded wheelchairs! Needless to say we ceased to use that particular taxi firm for the remainder of the holiday.

Individual support and leisure projects

Many projects providing leisure activities and outings for young disabled people are unable to offer individual support on request, as it is seen to stretch beyond their budget limitations. Such projects are in the main run by voluntary organisations that necessarily spend a great deal of time maintaining current funding. Few projects have secure core funding and consequently can rarely afford to offer young disabled people individual support to follow their own interests in their own communities. Young disabled people requiring individual support are therefore effectively denied access to such projects unless they can bring their own support with them.

Due to the general lack of support in mainstream leisure centres, youth clubs, etc., young people with impairments who require support to participate in activities can only access such venues when they are taken by their families or when they visit as part of a segregated group. Few of the voluntary projects providing leisure activities for young disabled people offer regular individual support to young people enabling them to go to places they choose to go to, at the time they choose. There is also little evidence of statutory agencies providing individual support allowing disabled young people to pursue their own chosen leisure interests. Such a general lack of provision plays a large part in the isolation of disabled young people requiring such support, as it can effectively deny them the right to be present in their communities.

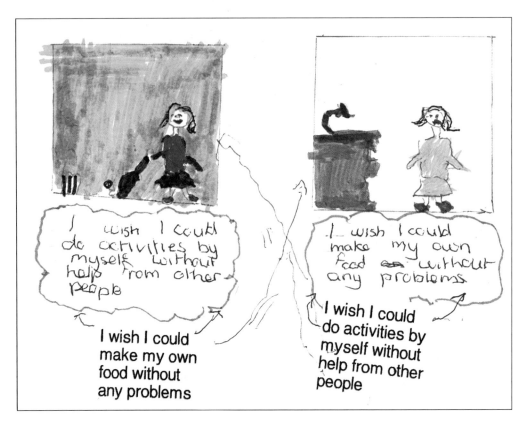

In a culture encouraging a rigid independence, Mita longs to do things on her own ...

Mita knows what she would like ...

Mita requires support to go out, to access transport, to take part in leisure activities such as swimming, bowling, etc. The type of support she requires might be described as 'little and often' – she needs an arm to balance on as she steps from the pavement onto the road; a hand to help her out of the swimming pool; a pair of hands to carry her food and drink in a cafe; or two people to help her get into a go-cart. The result of her not having this support is significant – some evenings and weekends she does little more than watch television as she can do this independently.
In a culture encouraging a rigid independence, Mita longs to do things on her own, although, in school, she has found her own acceptable ways of her support needs being met:

> *I am getting quite a lot of help at school. Recently I had decided to have no help in two of the lessons and right now my friend helps me in those lessons.*

Because of the way in which we, as a society, view teenage years as a time that young people have the right to be free from responsibilities towards each other, in addition to the way that impairment is viewed as an undesirable, extraordinary phenomenon, this very natural, supportive relationship between Mita and her friends does not appear to spread into relationships beyond the classroom.

Kevin knows what he wants ...

One young man taking part in this project desperately wants to be out doing all the things he sees his non-disabled peers doing. Kevin does not want to go to specialist clubs or holiday schemes. He wants to hang out in the places he sees other young people hanging out; he wants to be doing things and going places. Kevin's social services department provides him with three hours a week individual support, and this is currently under threat because he and his family are perceived to be 'coping'. Kevin enjoys going out with his support worker each week and looks forward to the time they spend together. He also wants to go out at other times. He wants to be able to go down to the local shops, to go to the park when he feels like it (as opposed to when an adult is available to take him), and he wants to hang out and chat to people he meets in the street. The fact that the support he requires to do these ordinary activities is not available presents a formidable barrier to his being present in his local community in the way in which he would choose, in addition to the consequent lack of opportunities to make and develop friendships.

Andrew knows what makes him happy ...

Andrew is another young man who likes to be out 'doing his own thing' – sometimes experiencing the freedom of large open spaces, at other times taking his support worker to places of his choosing.

Over the summer holidays, with several different people he knew and liked to support him, Andrew embarked on a variety of different activities, the first of which was a holiday camp for teenagers.

During his time at camp, Andrew chose which activities he would like to take part in. He was able to spend time with other young people or go off on his own. When Andrew and his support worker were established, other workers at the camp, seeing such a

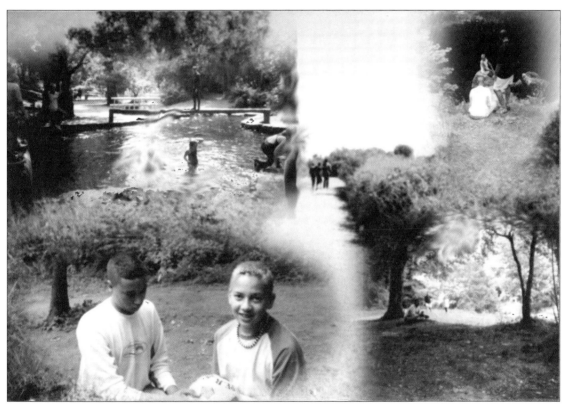

During his time at camp, Andrew chose which activities he would like to take part in.

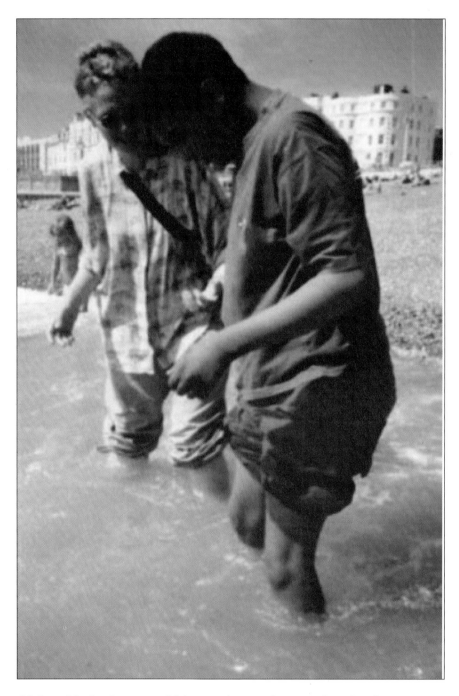

Although Andrew and his mother enjoy each other's company immensely, both of them enjoy the ordinary experience of doing things with other people from time to time.

positive relationship, offered to support Andrew for short periods. In this way, he had the experience of being 'one of many', of blending in with the crowd. The other young people present had the opportunity of seeing someone they perceived as 'different ' having an ordinary time, being part of the group.

In addition to time away from home with other young people, Andrew also went on days out and weekends away. With support of his choosing in place, he was able to access ordinary activities with someone other than his mother – his most frequent companion. Although Andrew and his mother enjoy each other's company immensely, both of them also enjoy the ordinary experience of doing things with other people from time to time.

There were several striking features of the relationship between Andrew and his support workers/personal assistants:

- Andrew knew, liked and felt comfortable with his support workers.

- The support workers enjoyed being with Andrew.

- The support workers were comfortable and confident about understanding Andrew's methods of communication and about their own ability to communicate with him.

- Occasionally, two support workers spent time together with Andrew. This not only provided them with support and confidence but also had the welcome side effect of lessening the intensity of the support relationship, making it more ordinary.

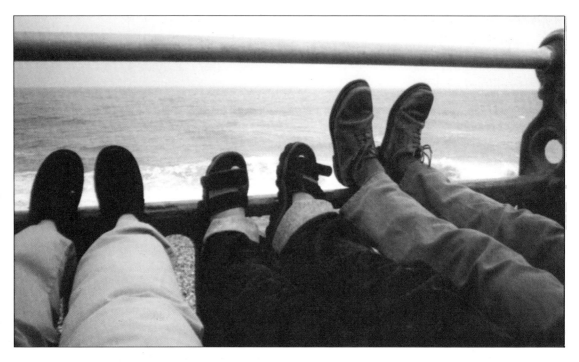

This … had the welcome side effect of lessening the intensity of the support relationship, making it more ordinary.

Things to think about …

The issues surrounding the provision of appropriate support are complex. One project, keen to enable disabled young people to go to a local disco, provided a support worker to go with them. Wanting to give the young people as ordinary an experience as possible, the support worker spent the night trying to be available and inconspicuous at the same time. Many young disabled people felt constrained by the constant presence of an adult in a supervisory capacity:

> *The biggest barrier is that I'm not allowed to go out on my own or with my friends. There is always an adult with us.*

'Hanging out' is a typical pastime of young people. The dynamics of hanging out change in the presence of an adult, it simply is not the same experience. Many disabled young people with high support needs have little opportunity to 'hang out'. In part this is due to the fact that they are likely to attend special schools and therefore their local peers have had little opportunity to learn how to be with them, how to support them or how to 'hang out' with them. A clear example of this can be found with those young people requiring individual support to communicate who have only experienced segregated provision:

> *… I am excluded from so much and I am so lonely and have few friends.*

This experience stands in sharp contrast to that of another young man who also requires support to communicate but who has always attended local mainstream schools (albeit on a part-time basis):

> Blake: *Good friends? Seven or eight good friends at school. Vinnie, good friend, go swimming. Chris not fazed.*

Mother: *Why not fazed?*

Blake: *Does not bother him.*

Mother: *What does not bother him?*

Blake: *Me.*

It is often said that it is not fair to ask young people to support each other, that it places too much responsibility on young shoulders. Young people taking part in this project were keen to spend time with each other and were asking for and giving support to one another in a natural way. When impairment is viewed as a natural part of our human experience, the support required and given becomes as ordinary as helping a friend.

Communication support

Several of the young people taking part in this project used 'facilitated communication', others used sign language to communicate, whilst others did not use any formal method of communication but expressed their preferences through their behaviour and/or their body. Whenever any one of these methods is a means of communication, the young person requires the presence of a facilitator either to support their communication or to interpret their wishes. None of the young people had any communication support outside of their educational setting and so had to rely on family or friends to take on the role of facilitating or interpreting their communication. These young people were therefore denied the opportunity to hang out with other young people, to develop 'ordinary' relationships, or to take part in ordinary leisure pursuits in the way in which the majority of young people do.

Support to facilitate friendships

Because the value of relationships to young disabled people perceived as having communication impairments, learning difficulties and/or high levels of support needs is not generally recognised, there is little acknowledgement that some young people require support to facilitate friendships. The majority of projects providing activities for young people perceived as having learning difficulties focus on activities rather than hanging out, being together, or building relationships. The lack of relationships between young disabled women perceived as having learning difficulties was particularly marked. Support workers (so often employed on a temporary, part-time basis) appeared to concentrate on involving these young women in activities rather than creating opportunities for them to cement friendships. Young people perceived as having learning difficulties, however, clearly conveyed that their priority was to develop relationships, make new friends and hang out with established friends. Activities were enjoyed and appreciated but did not appear to be the main event.

Financial support

The majority of young people taking part in this project were either at school or at college – only one young person was in full-time employment. It was notable that, in spite of including young people up to the age of 19 or 20, not one of the young people taking part had a weekend or holiday job. This is something that the majority of young non-disabled people have the opportunity to experience. Having no independent means of earning money threw the young people back on the resources of either their parents or welfare benefits. In this way, they lacked opportunities to begin to enjoy a small amount of financial independence and were excluded from an experience valued by the majority of teenagers.

Mutual support – sharing experiences

Many of the young people involved in this project, whilst wanting to be welcomed and included in mainstream leisure activities alongside non-disabled young people, attributed positive value to the existence of segregated clubs and holiday schemes. For Ben and Lizzie, the segregated leisure project in their home town had 'saved their lives'. It was to the friends they made at this project that they turned when they found themselves isolated in mainstream school. Having attended the project from an early age, it provided them with a natural base from which to build relationships with other young disabled children and teenagers. In their younger years, they enjoyed doing ordinary things in groups, facilitated by support workers, with other young disabled people. In their early teenage years, it was with friends made in the group that they were able to talk about their personal experience of discrimination and oppression. Sharing experiences with each other gave them the understanding that the problem did not lie with them as individuals but rather within a disabling society. In their later teenage years, they have developed independent relationships with each other that have enabled them to leave the project behind. This year a small group of friends from the project went on a week's holiday together in exactly the same way that many teenagers do. They planned the week together, made the appropriate arrangements and went off to have a very ordinary experience.

It is through ordinary relationships with each other that they have been able to explore their personal experiences of discrimination and oppression. Sharing experiences with each other has given them the understanding that the problem does not lie within them as individuals but rather within a disabling society. All members of this loose knit group have non-disabled friends, but it is to each other they turn when they encounter barriers to participating in the mainstream.

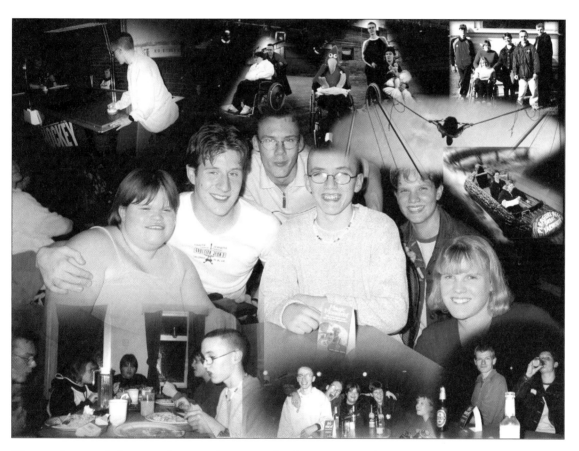

They planned the week together, made the appropriate arrangements and went off to have a very ordinary experience.

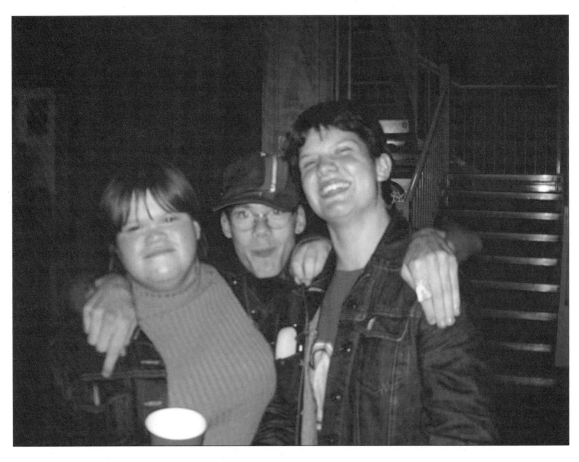

... it is to each other they turn when they encounter barriers to participating in the mainstream.

Similarly, Mita, Sally and James found that their confidence increased enormously after spending a week on an adventure holiday organised by the Royal National Institute for the Blind (RNIB). This week was specifically for young people with visual impairments attending mainstream school. Recognising both the dangers of isolation in this setting and specific training required by the young people to enable them to go out independently, the RNIB organises such holidays regularly. Many young people return year after year, stating that it not only increases their confidence but also gives them a break from their families.

Coming to Atlantic College means that I get some freedom and a rest from my mum. It allows me to try out sports like sand sledging and tobogganing, rope course and initiative games that I wouldn't be able to do at home. I get to meet new friends with the same problems I have. I had never been to Wales before so it gave me an opportunity to see a part of the country I had never seen before. I love having the thrill of new experiences and that's what these holidays provide.

Although there was little evidence of empowerment being an integral part of schemes run for disabled people with learning difficulties, there was evidence in some schemes of young people with learning difficulties having a good time together and, on rare occasions, of 'ordinary' relationships taking place between them.

The value and importance of having the opportunity to make ordinary relationships with other young people with similar impairments should not be overlooked. For the young people with other impairments, it was through such relationships that they were able to understand their experience. A notable feature of some groups providing leisure activities for young disabled people perceived as having learning difficulties was that the young people were more interested in forming relationships with non-disabled support workers (especially young support workers) than they were

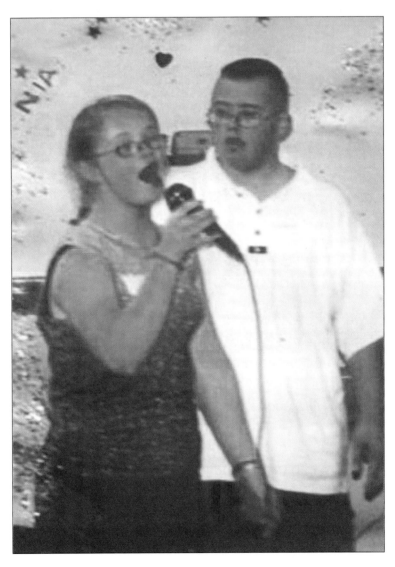

… on rare occasions, there was evidence of 'ordinary' relationships taking place between young people perceived as having learning difficulties.

with each other. Whilst this is not necessarily a bad thing, there is a danger that, without specific training for support workers on the subtleties of the barriers denying people perceived as having learning difficulties the right to mutually valued relationships, relationship dynamics whereby the young person with learning difficulties is treated as being 'incompetent' are likely to be in play.

In direct contradiction to the dominant view that to be 'autistic' means having no interest in developing relationships, Osian turns to the company of other young people perceived as being 'autistic' for mutual support and companionship:

I am excluded from so much and I am so lonely and have few friends apart from autistics who do not communicate with me using language but we feel an affinity which takes away isolation.

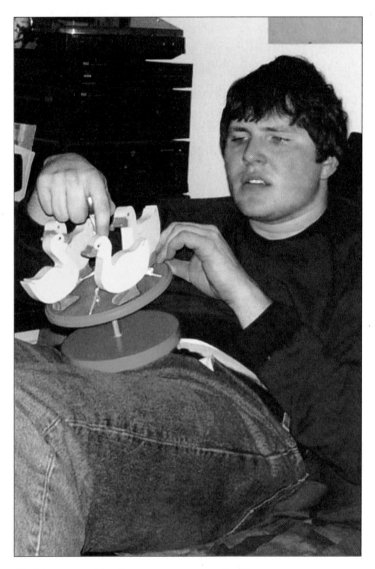

Osian turns to the company of other young people perceived as being autistic for mutual support and companionship.

9 Information

Disabled young people with a wide range of impairments showed that they knew what they liked doing, where they liked going and with whom they enjoyed spending their time. Many disabled young people taking part were able to identify the different barriers they faced to their inclusion within the mainstream. Markedly absent, however, was a general lack of information of ways in which they might follow through on their own ideas for breaking down disabling barriers. There was, for example, a notable lack of knowledge about Direct Payments – what they were, whether or not individuals were entitled to them and how to get them. Similarly, there was little knowledge about the existence of Independent Living Centres. As young people, their families and professionals working alongside them generally know very little about policy initiatives and consequent funding opportunities, the possibilities of placing young disabled people in a position of shaping their own futures, influencing the way services (mainstream and segregated) are delivered, are extremely limited. Without easily accessible, appropriate information, it is very difficult for young disabled people to begin to break down exclusive barriers.

The co-ordinator of a popular and successful holiday scheme run by a voluntary agency said that he thought many disabled teenagers in the city never got to hear about the scheme and were therefore denied the opportunity to take part. Those young people participating either knew about it through their social worker or because they happened to know someone else attending the scheme. Through these avenues, the scheme is always oversubscribed and so has no need to publicise its provision. One undesirable outcome of this is that the most isolated disabled young people (young people from minority ethnic backgrounds; those with the most complex impairments; and those within families living in poverty) are unlikely to ever hear about such schemes. Not knowing of their existence means that they will never request a place; this in turn means that their isolation increases.

How is information given?

Receiving information about schemes, activities, clubs and/or events is the first stage to being welcomed in those places. In order to make informed choices, we have to have information readily available. The experience of Andrew provides a reminder of the complexities involved in giving and receiving information. Andrew is unable to communicate directly that he would like to go to a certain place at a particular time. He is therefore dependent on those who know him well to take him to the places they know from experience he enjoys going to. Information given in the way of leaflets or advertisements is insufficient for Andrew to make informed choices. Andrew makes his wishes clear by taking people to the places he wants to go to. If he is to try out untested experiences, he has to have information about different possibilities. In a culture that widely perceives Andrew to be 'incompetent', it often comes as a surprise when he demonstrates a creative competency. On one occasion, as Andrew was going to one of his favourite places with two of his support workers, he sat in the back of the car apparently engrossed in his own thoughts, whilst his support workers talked about the possibility of going to the London Eye. They thought Andrew might like it but were reluctant to try it out as it was expensive and full of unknown quantities – 'What if he doesn't like it and we're stuck at the top?' They decided to stick to their original plan and take Andrew to a tried and tested venue – an amusement arcade. When the support workers parked the car near to the arcade, Andrew wandered off in the opposite direction and found his way to the front of the queue of the London Eye, support workers in tow. Having received the information, gleaned from the discussion in the car, he was able to make a clear choice about where he wanted to go.

Other young people, because of the nature of their impairment, are unable to make choices in this way. Hearing conversations may not be enough to allow them to make informed choices. Trying things out is sometimes the only way in which family, friends or support workers can ascertain whether the young person enjoys something or not. On occasion it is necessary to try things out several times to ascertain whether or not it is something the young person enjoys doing. 'Having a go' is often discounted as a means of giving information, as it is obviously expensive. For some young disabled people, however, it is the only way of making informed choices.

What will we find when we get there?

Information about the possibilities of going to different places, doing different things is not the only thing that is required. It is often necessary to know beforehand about issues of physical access. The availability of suitable toilets, changing facilities, seating arrangements, loop systems, concessionary prices for both the disabled person and the support worker/personal assistant, parking space, etc. are all important components in a decision to go to a particular place and can affect the experience of the visit. One project leader spent a day going round toilets and parking spaces on Oxford Street before taking a group of young disabled teenagers on a shopping expedition, as experience had taught her that the success of the day was dependent upon such research.

10 **Conclusion**

In all conversations with young disabled people on the subject of inclusive leisure, the emphasis has been on interdependence and the centrality of relationship. Whilst opportunities to try out a range of leisure activities and pursuits are appreciated, it is the opportunity to be in mutually valued relationships that young disabled people identify as the key to the possibility of their inclusion in mainstream culture. Whilst leisure provides a natural building ground for the development of relationships based on a common interest, placing such valued relationships in the mainstream allows discriminatory and oppressive attitudes to be broken down as natural enjoyment and positive relationships become visible to the public at large. In this way, leisure is seen as a key area through which to pave the way for a more inclusive society.

Opportunities for reciprocal relationship are dependent on opportunities to be present. Young disabled people perceived as having complex cognitive, sensory, physical and communication impairments are all too often denied this fundamental right. Educated in segregated schools with little or no support to be present in their local communities, the possibilities for engaging in reciprocal relationship with people of their choice are severely limited. Their continuing absence, whilst perpetuating the cultural values lying behind their experience of exclusion, demonstrates their denial of the right to relationship.

This baseline of exclusion for those young people perceived as 'being the most difficult to include' affects all young people. The experience of other disabled young people demonstrates that, although their presence may be tolerated, they can rarely rely on being welcomed. All too often disabled young people are either prevented or discouraged from participating in mainstream activities through physical, cultural, economical or psychological barriers.

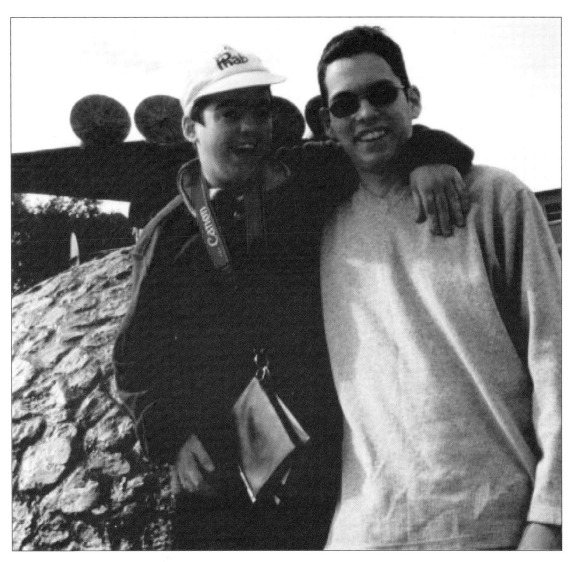

... it is the opportunity to be in mutually valued relationships that young disabled people identify as the key to the possibility of their inclusion to mainstream culture.

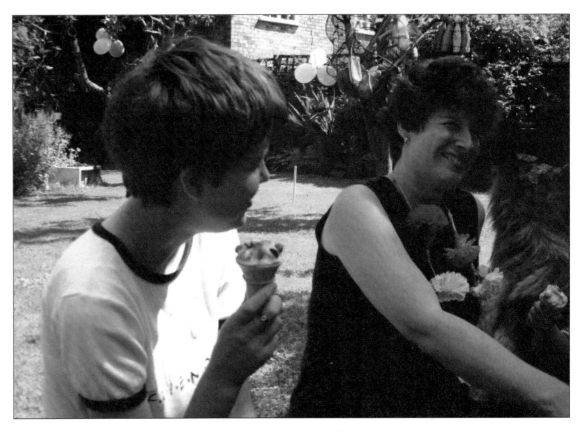

... the emphasis has been on interdependence and the centrality of relationship.

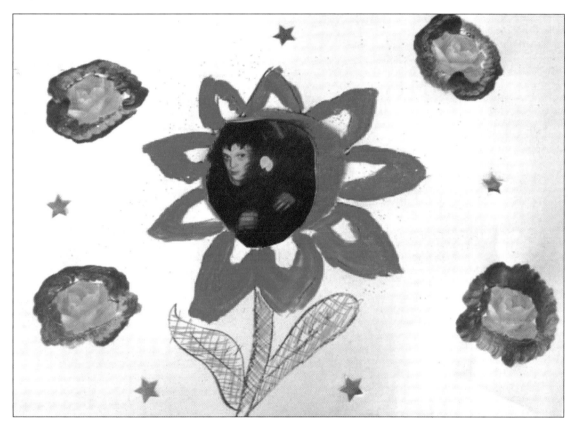

Opportunities for reciprocal relationship are dependent on opportunities to be present.

Throughout this project, in all of the conversations with young disabled people, it has been apparent that they have many ideas for ways in which their experience of exclusion can be transformed to one of inclusion. Their ideas range from enforcing present legislation (such as the Disability Discrimination Act) to improving the way we behave towards each other. In this sense, they are asking for change to come from all of us – not simply from politicians and service providers, but also from teachers, social workers, bus drivers, youth workers, project leaders, support workers, shopkeepers and people they meet on the street.

There is a great willingness from young disabled people both to talk about their experience and to engage with a process leading to change. They want to be able to tell others about their experiences, they want service providers (leisure, education, health and social services) to learn from them in order that their experience of exclusion ceases. In the present climate of consultation, young disabled people are asking for their views to be taken seriously. By asking to be listened to, they are asking us to act on what we hear in order to implement change, in whatever way we can, in whatever role we happen to be in. Practical change positively affecting their lives, individually and collectively, locally and nationally, is the measuring stick given for effective listening.

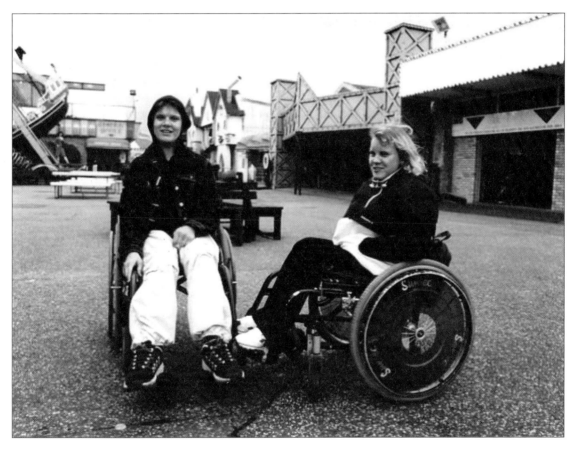

There is a great willingness from young disabled people both to talk about their experience and to engage with a process leading to change.

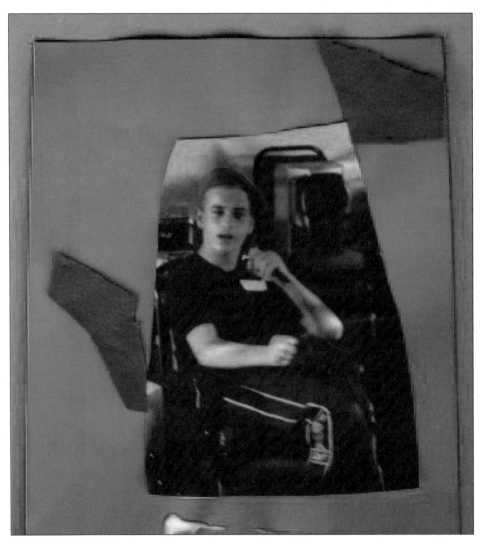

In the present climate of consultation, young disabled people are asking for their views to be taken seriously.

11 A note of caution …

Before considering recommendations arising from the experience of young disabled people, it is perhaps necessary to reflect for a moment on what they are saying. The main thrust of the message has been that the heart of inclusion lies within relationship. Whilst young disabled people have clearly identified a wide range of barriers to their full and equal participation in the mainstream, the emphasis on relationship indicates that the nature of change is necessarily a process rather than a 'one-off action' or an end result. It is, then, only when necessary physical change (for example, accessible transport) meets with attitudinal change (for example, impairment being viewed as ordinary) that 'inclusion' can be said to be in place. Within this process, there is a part for everyone – our interdependence means that, until we are all equally valued and included, the whole is not complete. The recommendations that follow in Chapter 12, therefore, are intended to be placed within this context. They do not stand alone, as 'things to be done', or 'boxes to be ticked', but rather are recognised as part of an intricate, ever creative process dependent on respectful, mutually reciprocal relationship.

12 Recommendations

A major source of frustration for young disabled people is based in the lack of 'bite' within the Disability Discrimination Act, 1995, lying alongside a perceived reluctance of service providers and the general public to 'take it on'. Young disabled people were largely unaware of policy initiatives (and the resulting funding opportunities) such as Children First and Quality Protects. Professionals within the voluntary sector were similarly unaware of such initiatives and therefore of the way in which they could be used to build on present service provision.

At the heart of such policy initiatives is the prerequisite for service providers to obtain the views of the young people for whom they are offering a service. This, in turn, lies within the larger context of the establishment of a new government department – the Children and Young Persons' Unit – that seeks to place the views of young people at the centre of policy development when that policy affects the lives of children and young people. As adults, we have much to learn about the way in which we listen to children and young people.

This is even more so when we, as predominantly non-disabled adults, listen to disabled children and young people. Listening to young disabled people is something we can all do, in whatever role we happen to be in.

Throughout this project, young disabled people have highlighted the importance of being in mutually reciprocal, valued relationships and the way in which we do not exist as independent units but, rather, are connected to each other. Creative use of these two themes provides the starting point for the implementation of change both locally and nationally. In putting forward recommendations for action, young disabled people are pointing to change on two fronts:

- on an interpersonal level (mutually valued relationships)

- on a wide societal level (for example: through the enforcement of the Disability Discrimination Act, 1995; the use of monies made available through different policy and funding initiatives; the translation of the rhetoric of legislation into the practicalities of everyday experience).

The onus is placed on all of us, in whatever role we happen to be in, to engage with the process of change. The following section gives ideas for ways in which change, based on the themes given by young disabled people, might be achieved. This list is not intended to be comprehensive as the potential for change lying within relationship is a continual process of discovery. It is hoped that the central message of this report allows for professionals in a wide range of areas (education, leisure, social services, health and the voluntary sector) and working at different levels (youth workers, planners, policy makers nationally and locally, development workers, voluntary and statutory workers, teachers, social workers, leisure service personnel and so on) to explore their own way of affecting change alongside the young disabled people they seek to serve.

Young disabled people

Perhaps the most important recommendation to come from this report is also the simplest. The starting point for meaningful change in the experience of young disabled people has to come from those young people themselves. Although they have offered many practical ideas for change, the basis they give is that of being valued and respected. We do not necessarily have to set up special projects to listen to young disabled people; we can listen in whatever capacity we happen to be in, allow relationships to develop and move forwards together. Within this context, the following specific projects are recommended:

- further research projects that seek to find out and disseminate the views of young disabled people, recognise the importance of and develop opportunities for 'being present'

- specific projects dedicated to examining the barriers to both the expression of and the listening to the views of young disabled people perceived as having learning difficulties

- local and national networking opportunities recognising the benefit of sharing experiences with other young disabled people whilst also acknowledging the need for disabled and non-disabled young people to have the chance to build positive relationships (networking possibilities are enormous with the use of the World Wide Web, email and telephone texting)

- the inclusion of young disabled people in the development and delivery of training packages and as members of management committees/advisory boards.

Including the families of young disabled people

There is presently a tension for young disabled people and their families in the way in which their family relationships are perceived. The predominant view that impairment is something to be fixed, denied and shied away from often masks the fact that relationships between young disabled people and other family members are completely ordinary. To this end, suggestions for future research and publications include projects seeking to:

- make visible positive family relationships

- explore the tension for parents around apparently conflicting issues of empowerment and protection

- evaluate the effect the provision of appropriate support to participate in mainstream leisure provision has on the family experience and requests for 'respite care'

- develop opportunities for parents, brothers and sisters to be involved in the development of training packages and as members of management committees/advisory boards

- include the views of non-disabled sisters and brothers alongside those of disabled young people.

Dissemination of good practice

Just as there is much isolation for disabled young people, so, too, are projects running in isolation from each other. At present, new groups are not always benefiting from the experience of established groups.

- The development of the national co-ordination of information on progressive leisure opportunities in both voluntary and statutory agencies. Such information to be made easily available to disabled children and young people, families, professionals in statutory and voluntary sector and policy makers through a co-ordinated web project.

- The development of local and national networking opportunities for project development workers, support staff and youth workers in both segregated and mainstream provision.

Education

In light of the fact that young disabled people highlighted their educational experience as key to their leisure experience, the following section makes some suggestions for work within the educational setting (school and/or college). This work does not have to be done on a 'grand scale' but rather is suggested as work to be done on a smaller, local scale, building on existing opportunities within the curriculum.

- Research projects based in schools seeking to build on existing good practice around the building of relationships between disabled and non-disabled young people.

- Research projects exploring:
  1. the experience of having a support worker in the school setting
  2. the identification of good practice around facilitating friendships.

- Schools to engage with pupils about access needs such as classroom materials (large-print books) and necessary physical adaptations (painting the edge of the stairs in a bright colour), and local education authorities to release funding to arrange for such access needs to be met.

Information

All too often, disabled young people and their families appear to be learning about leisure opportunities through word of mouth. This means that those young people with the best networks are the ones making use of the very limited resources available. There is a need for the giving of information to be recognised as part of the process of inclusion in that it provides the first step to being welcomed into facilities, services and resources.

- Local authorities to produce leaflets advertising present accessible leisure provision in a range of formats including: different languages (depending on local ethnic groups); large print; Braille; pictures and symbols.

- The development (and advertisement) of free taster sessions for disabled young people (and their support workers if necessary) recognised and made available as a means of giving information about activities.

- Research projects to uncover ways of reaching the most
  excluded groups of young disabled people and to monitor the
  effect of targeted information dissemination to such groups.

Multi-agency initiatives

The process of working towards the provision of leisure services
that welcome and include all young people necessitates the
coming together of different agencies in both the voluntary and the
statutory sectors. The way in which disabled young people link
their leisure experience with other aspects of their lives
demonstrates the way in which services impinge upon one another.
For example, the existence of a welcoming leisure centre, where
appropriate support is provided, is undermined if young people
cannot easily access public transport.

- In recognition of the leading role played by voluntary agencies
  in the provision of leisure services through holiday schemes,
  out-of-school clubs, youth clubs, etc., core funding to be made
  available to such groups via their local authorities. In addition to
  this core funding, more flexible funding arrangements to be
  made available as necessary to allow for flexibility in the
  employment of support staff.

- Project development work between voluntary agencies, social
  services, leisure services, education departments and health
  services placing leisure central to the lives of young disabled
  people.

Support

The provision of appropriate support is of vital importance as it
brings together the central issues identified by disabled young
people: reciprocal relationship and interdependence. The provision
and development of appropriate support allows for the exploration

of ways in which environments can welcome young disabled people in addition to providing examples of mutually enjoyable relationships.

- The development of evaluation and research projects, through the statutory and the voluntary sector, to explore ways in which young disabled people choose to be supported in their time out of school, college or work.

- The promotion of Direct Payments as a means of accessing support to participate in leisure activities of choice.

- Social services, leisure services and voluntary agencies to work together to provide support in a range of venues as an alternative to traditional 'respite care'.

- Development projects based in leisure centres and other public facilities to help staff routinely identify the support needs of their client groups as part of their role as workers in the public services.

- Identification and recognition of use of informal support networks.

- Research and development projects to explore the support offered through the development of 'ordinary relationships' between disabled and non-disabled young people.

- The role of voluntary care agencies (e.g. Leonard Cheshire) in the provision of support.

- Free entrance to the use of facilities when in the role of support worker/personal assistant.

Training

The majority of voluntary projects provided their own 'disability awareness' or 'disability equality' training to both their own staff and on occasion to staff of local leisure service providers. There is little guidance or monitoring of such training with regard to content, delivery, or effectiveness. Projects were therefore providing training around disability issues without clear guidelines and/or the benefit of existing training developed and offered by disabled adults. In order to develop existing good practice in voluntary agencies providing leisure services for young disabled people, there is a specific need for:

- funding to be made available, locally and nationally, for the development of standardised disability equality training, developed and delivered by disabled adults and young people, to project development workers, youth workers and support workers, alongside front-line staff in both social and leisure services.

And finally ... back to relationship

As part of this project, two young men (Blake and Osian) who communicate through facilitated communication 'talked' with each other about their experience of leisure. In keeping with all other young people taking part, the conversation covered all aspects of their lives – what they liked doing, education, exams, future prospects, friendships and music. In response to being asked what his favourite music was, Blake promptly replied, 'Destiny's Child, "I'm a survivor"'. Asked why this was his favourite, Blake replied:

We survive. You, me, everybody ...

A week or so later, I happened to hear the song being played on the radio. Curious to find out why it appealed so strongly to Blake, I listened carefully to the words of the song:

I'm a survivor
I'm gonna make it ...

The words are a reflection not only of his positivity, but also that of the majority of disabled young people taking part in this project. In spite of lives dominated by the experience of exclusion, they are naturally and spontaneously, through reciprocal relationship, offering the rest of us opportunities to build bridges of understanding, leading the way towards an inclusive society. The question is not so much whether they will make it, but whether the rest of us will keep up with them.

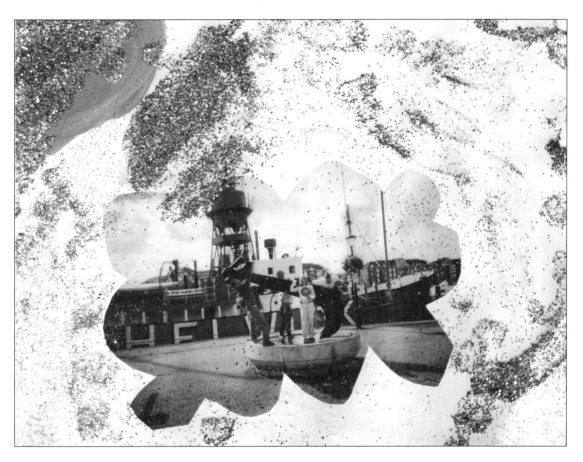

Goodbye, but not farewell …

References

Aitchison, C. (2000) *Disability and Social Inclusion: Leisure, Sport and Culture in the Lives of Young Disabled People*. Cheltenham and Gloucester: College of Higher Education

HMSO (2001) *Valuing People: A New Strategy for Learning Disability for the 21st Century*. London: The Stationery Office

MacKeith, M. (2000) 'Maresa's inside story', in P. Murray and J. Penman (eds) *Telling Our Own Stories – Reflections on Family Life in a Disabling World*. Sheffield: Parents with Attitude

Petrie, P., Egharevba, I., Oliver, C. and Poland, G. (2000) *Out of School Lives, Out of School Services*. London: The Stationery Office

Sellin, B. (1995) *In Dark Hours I Find My Way – Messages from an Autistic Mind*. London: Victor Gollancz

Useful reading list

This list makes no claims to be comprehensive. Hopefully, it provides a starting point for both learning about new initiatives and providing networking opportunities.

An Easy Guide to Direct Payments. London: Department of Health. (Available from DOH Publications, PO Box 777, London SE1 6XH. Email: doh@prologistics.co.uk Website: www.doh.gov.uk/directp.htm)

BT Countryside for All – A Good Practice Guide to Disabled People's Access in the Countryside. (Available from The Fieldfare Trust, 67a The Wicker, Sheffield, South Yorkshire or through its website: www.fieldfare.org.uk)

Cole-Hamilton, Issy and Vale, Dan (2000) *Shaping the Future: The Experiences of Blind and Partially Sighted Children in the UK*. London: Royal National Institute for the Blind

Disability Discrimination Act 1995 – Code of Practice: Rights of Access; Goods, Facilities, Services and Premises. London: The Stationery Office. (Available from The Publications Centre, PO Box 276, London SW8 5DT. Telephone: 0870 600 5522)

Edinburgh and East of Scotland Deaf Society (2002) *Access All Areas – A Report on Access to Social, Cultural and Leisure Activities for Young Deaf People*. Edinburgh: Edinburgh and East of Scotland Deaf Society. (Available from the Edinburgh and East of Scotland Deaf Society, 49 Albany Street, Edinburgh EH1 3QY. Telephone: 0131 556 3128 [voice]; 0131 557 0419 [text]. Fax: 0131 557 82830)

Finch, Naomi, Lawton, Dot, Williams, Julie and Sloper, Patricia (2000) *Disability Survey 2000: Survey of Young Disabled People and Sport.* York: Social Policy Research Unit, University of York. (Available from Sport England, Information Centre, 16 Upper Woburn Place, London WCIH 0QP. Enquiry line: 0207 273 1700)

Keil, Sue (2001) *Shaping the Future: Life and Leisure Activities of Blind and Partially Sighted Children and Young People Aged 5–25.* London: Royal National Institute for the Blind

Planning Individual Leisure Activities for Adults with Visual and Learning Disabilities. Royal National Institute for the Blind Focus and Factsheet. (Available from RNIB Customer Services, PO Box 173, Peterborough PE2 6WS. Telephone: 0845 702 3153)

The Inclusion Assistant. A booklet and video about young people with high level support needs in mainstream schools. £10.00 (incl. P&P). (Available from Disability Equality in Education, Unit 4Q, Leroy House, 436 Essex Road, London N1 3QP)

Resource list

Again, this list makes no claims to be comprehensive but provides a starting point for an exploration of resources available, existing projects and opportunities for networking.

Access to the countryside
The Fieldfare Trust
67a The Wicker
Sheffield
South Yorkshire
Telephone: 0114 270 1668
Fax: 0114 276 7900
Minicom: 0114 275 5380
Website: www.fieldfaretrust.org.uk
Email: Fieldfare@BTInternet.com

The Fieldfare Trust promotes access to the countryside and environmental education for disabled people

Sporting organisations

Sport England
16 Upper Woburn Place
London WC1H 0QP
Telephone: 020 7273 1700
Email: info@sportengland.org
Website: www.sportengland.org

English Federation of Disability Sport
Head Office
Manchester Metropolitan University
Alsager Campus
Hassall Road
Alsagar
Stoke-on-Trent ST7 2HL
Telephone: 0161 247 5294
Website: www.efds.co.uk

There is a network of ten regions that support national priorities and develop sports programmes to respond to local needs. Details of local initiatives, such as the 'Inclusive Sports Club Programme', are available on the website. Also available on the website are details of publications including: *Including Disabled Pupils in PE; A Brighter Sporting Future for Disabled People; Coaching Disabled Footballers; and Millennium Festival Awards for All – Sport & Disability – A Simple Guide for Applicants.*

Inclusive Fitness Initiative
Thorncliffe Park Estate
Chapeltown
Sheffield S35 2PH
Telephone: 0114 257 2060
Website: www.efds.co.uk/regular/initfit.htm

This recent initiative aims to provide: the availability of inclusive fitness equipment; disability awareness/fitness training for fitness facility and front-of-house personnel; and the production of marketing and sports development packages that can be used to encourage, support and give access to various sporting opportunities to disabled people.

Arts and culture

Arts Council of England
14 Great Peter Street
London SW1P 3WQ
Telephone: 020 7333 0100 or 020 7973 6517
Website: www.artscouncil.org.uk

The Arts Council has produced several useful leaflets: *Disability Discrimination Act 1995 and the Arts; Arts Organisations and Rights of Access to Goods, Facilities and Services – Part III of the Disability Discrimination Act 1995;* and *The Disability Discrimination Act 1995 and the Arts.*These leaflets are available (free) from the Arts Council.

Artsline (London arts information service for disabled people)
54 Chalton Street
London NW1 1HS
Telephone: 020 7388 2227
Website: www.artsline.org.uk

Artsline offers a free telephone information service supplying detailed access information on theatres, cinemas, tourist attractions, selected restaurants and comedy and music venues. In addition, Artsline produces a range of access guides – details of publications are available on its website.

National Disability Arts Forum
Mea House
Ellison Place
Newcastle upon Tyne NE1 8XS
Telephone: 0191 261 1628
Website: www.ndaf.org.uk

The Forum promotes and supports the development of disability arts from local to international levels, and working with arts and other organisations in developing accessible arts environments.

The Forums provide help and advice on making organisations accessible to disabled people. The national Forum will tell you if there is a Forum local to you and how to contact them.

Learning Disability Arts Network for London
Website: www.networklondon.org.uk

A collection of artists in the London area who have learning difficulties or who work with and for people with learning difficulties. It includes workers in dance, drama, film, music, multi-media, video and the visual arts. The Network provides performances, presentations and workshops.

Heart 'n Soul
The Deptford Albany
Douglas Way
London SE8 4AG
Telephone: 020 8694 1632
Website: www.heartnsoul.co.uk

Heart 'n Soul is an arts organisation offering creative opportunities to people with learning difficulties. Activities include touring performances, clubs, training, residencies and workshops, providing opportunities for people with learning disabilities to realise their talents and personal potential.

Oily Cart
Smallwood School Annex
Smallwood Road
London SW17 0TW
Telephone: 020 8672 6329
Website: www.oilycart.org.uk

Oily Cart is a theatre company, based in London, which tours nationally with two new theatre productions each year: one for very young children, the other for young people with severe learning difficulties.

Equata
22 Lower Town
Sampford Peverell
Devon EX16 7BJ
Telephone: 01884 829265
Website: www.eclipse.co.uk/artshare

Equata is an organisation of disabled people which promotes
equality and access within the arts, primarily in South West
England. Equata aims to work alongside existing arts resources to
develop an inclusive arts environment – where disabled artists and
individuals have equal opportunities to produce, participate, plan
and manage arts projects and products.

Orpheus Centre
North Park Lane
Godstone
Surrey RH7 6HF
Telephone: 01883 744664
Website: www.orpheus.org.uk

The Orpheus Centre offers opportunities for disabled and non-
disabled people of all ages to develop skills in the performing arts.
Short courses (three-day and six-day) are offered as well as one-
to three-year apprenticeships, where young people can live and
work at the Centre.

Anjali Dance Company
Mill Cottage
The Mill Arts Centre
Spiceball Park
Banbury
Oxfordshire OX16 8QE
Telephone/fax: 01295 251909
Website: www.anjali.co.uk
Email: info@anjali.co.uk

Anjali Dance Company is a professional contemporary dance company. All dancers in the company have learning difficulties. The company produces and tours performances, and undertakes educational and outreach work.

Blue Eyed Soul
Belmont Arts Centre
5 Belmont
Shrewsbury SY1 1TE
Telephone: 01743 245998
Website: www.blueyedsoul.freeserve.co.uk
Email: admin@blueyedsoul.freeserve.co.uk

Working closely with local and national agencies on developing policy, training and performance opportunities, Blue Eyed Soul seeks to have an equal number of physically disabled and non-disabled members. Performances and workshops are offered.

Organisations

Dynamix Ltd
14 Montpelier Terrace
Mount Pleasant
Swansea SA1 6JW
South Wales
Telephone/fax: 01792 466231
Website: www.seriousfun.demon.co.uk
Email: Dynamix@seriousfun.demon.co.uk

Dynamix offers training and workshops within education, health, social services, charities and private businesses looking at a range of issues under the umbrella of social inclusion. Dynamix gives workshops on how to include young people with learning difficulties often considered 'too difficult to include' using a range of different media including music, multi-sensory techniques and 'serious fun'.

Edinburth Youth Inclusion Social Partnership
Unit 6
Castlecliff Workshops
25 Johnstone Terrace
Edinburgh EH1 2NH
Telephone: 0131 225 7388
Website: www.youthinclusion.org
Email: edinburgh@youthinclusion.org

Edinburgh Youth Social Inclusion Partnership runs a wide range of projects, working with organisations and young people to develop and test solutions for inclusion through action research, and promote their lasting implementation in good practice and policy development.

Disability Equality in Education
Unit 4Q
Leroy House
436 Essex Road
London N1 3QP
Telephone: 0207 359 2855
Website: www.diseed.org.uk
Email: info@diseed.org.uk

Provides training and resources for schools, colleges and local education authorities around the issue of inclusion for all students within our education system.

Parents for Inclusion
Unit 2
70 South Lambeth Road
London SW8 1RL
Telephone: 0207 582 5008 (helpline) and 0207 735 7735 (main office)
Website: www.parentsforinclusion.org

A national organisation of parents for parents, working with disabled people to ensure access to mainstream education for disabled children.

Young and Powerful
c/o Unit 2
70 South Lambeth Road
London SW8 1RL
Email: youngandpowerful@btinternet.com

A group of disabled and non-disabled young people who fight for the right to have their friendships, especially in schools, supported, so that they can support each other.

Alliance for Inclusive Education
Unit 2
70 South Lambeth Road
London SW8 1RL
Telephone: 0207 735 5277
Website: www.allfie.org.uk
Email: info@allfie.org.uk

A national campaigning organisation led by disabled people. Based on a network of individuals, families and groups working together, the Alliance wishes to bring about changes based on the conviction that all young people need to be educated in a single mainstream education system which can support young people to learn, play and live with each other.

National Centre for Independent Living
250 Kennington Lane
London SE11 5RD
Telephone: 0207 7857 1663
Website: www.bcodp.org.uk/ncil
Email: ncil@ncil.demon.co.uk

Provides information and advice on Direct Payments for personal
assistants to local authorities and supports the development of new
personal assistant support schemes.